OPERATIONS THAT MADE HISTORY

Second Edition

OPERATIONS THAT MADE HISTORY

Second Edition

Harold Ellis
C.B.E., D.M., M.Ch., F.R.C.S.
Emeritus Professor of Surgery, University of London

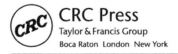

CRC Press
Taylor & Francis Group
Boca Raton London New York

CRC Press is an imprint of the
Taylor & Francis Group, an **informa** business

CRC Press
Taylor & Francis Group
6000 Broken Sound Parkway NW, Suite 300
Boca Raton, FL 33487-2742

© 2019 by Taylor & Francis Group, LLC
CRC Press is an imprint of Taylor & Francis Group, an Informa business

International Standard Book Number-13: 978-0-367-00155-1 (Hardback)
978-1-138-33431-1 (Paperback)

Library of Congress Cataloging-in-Publication Data

Names: Ellis, Harold, 1926- author.
Title: Operations that made history / Harold Ellis.
Description: Second edition. | Boca Raton, FL : CRC Press, [2018] | Includes bibliographical references and index.
Identifiers: LCCN 2018030132| ISBN 9781138334311 (pbk. : alk. paper) | ISBN 9780367001551 (hardback : alk. paper) | ISBN 9780429434280 (ebook)
Subjects: | MESH: General Surgery--history | Famous Persons | Surgical Procedures, Operative--methods | Case Reports
Classification: LCC RD19 | NLM WO 11.1 | DDC 617.092/2--dc23
LC record available at https://lccn.loc.gov/2018030132

Visit the Taylor & Francis Web site at
http://www.taylorandfrancis.com

and the CRC Press Web site at
http://www.crcpress.com

To my wife Wendy,
Our children and
grandchildren

CONTENTS

Part III   Famous Patients

INTRODUCTION

What constitutes an historic operation? Being a didactic under-graduate professor, I cannot help but answer this question by attempting a classification of the subject. After much study, I have divided such operations into Ellis type I, type II and type III.

Type I is the obvious group – the operation that today's newspapers love to describe as a 'major breakthrough' – the success never achieved before – the first gastrectomy, or pneumonectomy, or heart transplant. As an important rider to this it is usually, but not always, necessary for the operation to be not only original but also successful. Again and again throughout medical history there have been one or more unsung assays into something new, with fatal consequences, followed by the first loudly publicised success. Both the unsuccessful pioneer surgeon and his unfortunate dead patient pass into relative obscurity, in contrast to the worldwide acclaim of the victor. The unsuccessful gastrectomies of Jules Péan and Ludwig Rydigier are known only to the connoisseurs of medical history, but every medical student is familiar with the name of Theodor Billroth, whose gastrectomy in 1881 had that important qualification for an Ellis type I famous operation – his patient survived.

The Ellis type II operation may be insignificant in itself but marks the introduction of some important point in surgical technique. The best example of this was the removal, in 1846, of a fairly trivial cyst of the neck, which qualifies for its historic importance because it was the first demonstration by William T.G. Morton of ether anaesthesia. Another example was the first drainage of an axillary abscess by means of a tube drain. The surgeon was Lord Joseph Lister, and the patient happened to be Queen Victoria; as far as I know, she did not give informed consent for this experiment.

The type III operation depends entirely on the patient. The operation itself may be quite routine, and it is unusual, except in the example just given, for any important advance in technique to premiere at such an occasion. However, the fact that the surgeon's victim is famous rouses international interest. The majority of patients undergoing surgery for Crohn's disease go unnoticed, but if the intestine happens to belong to President Eisenhower, then diagrams of his alimentary tract are syndicated in newspapers throughout the world.

For the practising surgeon, perhaps most is learned from study of the type III cases. Certainly they teach an important lesson in how to deal with famous patients. In 1910, when young Bertie Dawson of the London Hospital (later Lord Dawson of Penn) was called to join the team looking after Edward VII, dying of cor pulmonale and chronic bronchitis, His Majesty asked the young man how he proposed to treat him. 'Sire', replied Dawson, 'I shall give you the best treatment possible. I shall treat you like any of my patients in the wards at the London Hospital'.

The lesson seems to be quite clear; any deviation from the norm may well lead to disaster. In 1923, when Sigmund Freud consulted his old friend Marcus Hajek with a carcinoma of his palate, the biopsy was carried out in a rather offhanded manner in the outpatient clinic. There was considerable bleeding; he had to be kept in overnight; further haemorrhage took place; the bedside bell was out of order, and the only thing that saved the great man's life was the prompt action of a cretinous dwarf in the other bed who rushed out and managed to get help. It is much wiser, in dealing with a VIP or a colleague, to take all the precautions that one usually adopts in dealing with more routine patients.

Famous patients appear rather braver than the norm and tend also to be very courteous. King George IV, after having his sebaceous cyst removed in 1821, without, of course, the benefit of any anaesthetic, said to Astley Cooper, 'What do you call these tumours?' To which Cooper replied, using the old Latin name, 'We call them steatomas, Sire'. 'Then', said the King, 'I hope this one will stay at home and not bother me again'. When Queen Victoria had her very unpleasant axillary abscess drained by Lister at Balmoral Castle in 1871, at fifty-one years of age, she said as she recovered from the chloroform, 'A most unpleasant task, Professor Lister, most pleasantly performed'. Very few less famous patients could express gratitude so charmingly.

Of course the rewards for performing an historic operation are great, but failure must be a bitter pill indeed, though not as serious now as in the days of Blind King John of Bohemia, who had all his surgeons drowned in the Danube when they failed to restore his sight.

Harold Ellis
London, England

Part I

MAJOR BREAKTHROUGHS

1

THE FIRST OVARIOTOMY

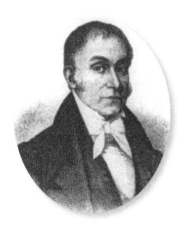

From time to time, I ask a new entry of medical students if they can guess the date of the first successful elective laparotomy, the name of the surgeon who performed the operation, and where it took place. After a long and profound silence, someone will tentatively suggest 'around 1870', guess at some well-known name, such as Joseph Lister (who, in fact, never opened the abdomen in his life), and opine that the venue must have been a London teaching hospital or one of the great European surgical clinics. None of these could be further from the truth, and I often surprise the class when I tell them that the date was 1809, the surgeon Ephraim McDowell, and the place Danville, Kentucky (Figure 1.1).

McDowell was the great-grandson of a Northern Irish Protestant who emigrated to the United States. His grandfather was killed in an Indian ambush; his father was a colonel in the Revolutionary War.

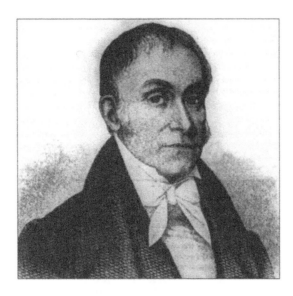

Figure 1.1 **Ephraim McDowell.** (Courtesy of the Royal College of Obstetricians and Gynaecologists, London.)

Our hero was born in Virginia in 1771 but moved to Kentucky at thirteen years of age when his father was appointed a judge at Danville, the first capital of that state, having 'upwards of 150 homes and some tolerably good buildings'. McDowell was apprenticed to study medicine with Dr Alexander Humphreys before going to Edinburgh, where he attended the sessions of 1793 and 1794, following the anatomy lectures of Alexander Munro (secundus) and studying surgery under John Bell. By 1795, he was back in Danville as its only surgeon. He soon built up an extensive practice covering hundreds of miles of frontier country; here a call meant a long ride on horseback in country where Indians and wolves were still a threat.

On December 13, 1809, McDowell was called to see Mrs Jane Todd Crawford, aged forty-four, who lived with her family in a log cabin at Motley's Glen, Green County, some distance from Danville (Figure 1.2). McDowell wrote:

> ...for several months [Mrs Crawford] thought herself pregnant. She was affected with pains similar to labour pains, from which

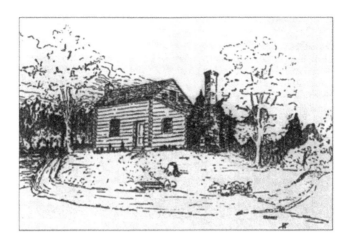

Figure 1.2 **The Crawford cabin in Green County, Kentucky.** (Reprinted with permission from Schachner A. *Ephraim McDowell: Father of Ovariotomy and Founder of Abdominal Surgery.* Philadelphia, JB Lippincott, 1921.)

she could find no relief. So strong was the presumption of her being in the last stage of pregnancy that two physicians, who were consulted on her case, requested my aid in delivering her. The abdomen was considerably enlarged and had the appearance of pregnancy, though the inclination of the tumour was to one side, admitting of an easy removal to the other. Upon examination per vaginam, I found nothing in the uterus, which induced the conclusion that it must be an enlarged ovarium... I gave to the unhappy woman information of her dangerous situation. She appeared willing to undergo an experiment, which I promised to perform if she would come to Danville (the town where I live), a distance of sixty miles from her place of residence.

McDowell could hardly have imagined that he would ever see his patient again, since such a journey 'appeared almost impracticable by any, even the most favourable conveyance'. However, Mrs Crawford was a tough frontier woman, and a few days later she appeared at his home in Danville, having made the difficult and dangerous journey by horseback. Interestingly enough, when the incision was made later in the abdominal wall,

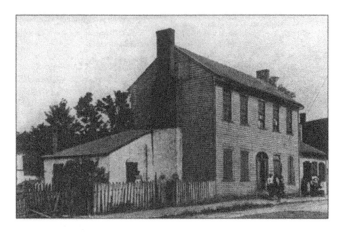

Figure 1.3 **The house in which Ephraim McDowell performed the first ovariotomy; this house is now carefully preserved and restored as a museum.** (Courtesy of the Royal College of Obstetricians and Gynaecologists, London.)

'the parietes were a good deal contused, which we ascribed to the resting of the tumour on the horn of the saddle during her journey'.

At this time, Ephraim's nephew, Dr James McDowell, who had graduated a few months before in Philadelphia, joined the practice as a partner. The young man made frequent attempts to dissuade his senior partner from operating. However, both McDowell and Mrs Crawford were determined on the experiment, and the operation was duly performed using the simplest of instruments, with no skilled help, in the front room of his home (Figure 1.3); naturally this was all carried out without any anaesthesia. Mrs Crawford recited psalms during the twenty-five minute ordeal, which took place on a Sunday – not just any Sunday, but Christmas Day. McDowell describes the operation (Figure 1.4) as follows:

Having placed her on a table of the ordinary height, on her back, and removed all her dressing which might in any way impede the operation, I made an incision about three inches from the musculus rectus abdominis, on the left side, continuing the same nine inches in length, parallel with the fibres of the above-named muscle, extending into the cavity

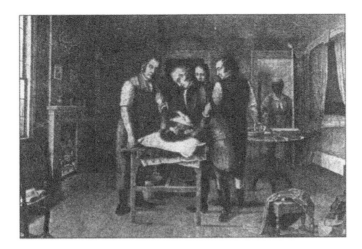

Figure 1.4 **'The First Ovariotomy', painted by George Knapp.** (Reprinted with permission from Schachner A. *Ephraim McDowell: Father of Ovariotomy and Founder of Abdominal Surgery.* Philadelphia, JB Lippincott, 1921.)

of the abdomen....The tumour then appeared full in view, but was so large that we could not take it away entire. We put a strong ligature around the Fallopian tube near the uterus, and then cut open the tumour, which was the ovarium and fimbrious part of the Fallopian tube very much enlarged. We took out 15 lbs of a dirty gelatinous-looking substance, after which we cut through the Fallopian tube and extracted the sac, which weighed 7 lbs and one-half. As soon as the external opening was made the intestines rushed out upon the table, and so completely was the abdomen filled by the tumour that they could not be replaced during the operation, which was terminated in about 25 minutes. We then turned her upon her left side, so as to permit the blood to escape, after which we closed the external opening with the interrupted suture, leaving out at the lower end of the incision the ligature which surrounded the Fallopian tube.

Within five days Mrs Crawford was up and about making her own bed, and in twenty-five days she returned home in good health by the same means as she came.

McDowell did not immediately publish this triumphant result – the first elective laparotomy successfully carried out for an accurately diagnosed intra-abdominal pathology. Perhaps he was too diffident, or perhaps he did not realise the tremendous implications of the case; possibly his busy practice gave him little time for the niceties of writing, and he was certainly not a particularly literary man. Most likely he realised that a comparatively unknown country surgeon, publishing a single case report, might be ridiculed unless further 'experiments' were attempted. Whatever the reason, McDowell waited until he had performed two further successful operations, both on black women, in 1813 and 1816, before publishing a report in 1817 of all three successes. His report appeared in the seventh volume of the *Eclectic Repertory and Analytical Review*, published in Philadelphia. Two years later, McDowell's second contribution appeared in the same journal, reporting two further cases, again both black women. One was successful, but the second patient died of peritoneal inflammation on the third post-operative day. Although McDowell published no more, he did continue with his experiments. Between 1822 and 1826, he operated on three more women, all of whom were white. In one, the ovarian mass was incised and drained, and the patient lived for a considerable period of time. One operation involved complete excision, and the third had to be abandoned at laparotomy due to extensive adhesions. There is evidence from correspondence that McDowell performed at least twelve operations for ovarian pathology, but no details exist of the later cases.

It certainly took some time for McDowell's successes to be accepted by the establishment (Figure 1.5). A copy of the 1817 report was sent to his old teacher, John Bell, in Edinburgh, who was then in Rome, where he died shortly thereafter; thus, John Lizars, who later became Professor of Surgery at the College of Surgeons of Edinburgh, received the report. Lizars did nothing about the paper until his own publication, *Observations on Extraction of Diseased Ovaria*, published in 1825, in which he reported four cases, one of which was successful in February 1825. In his report, he quoted McDowell's paper, although by now two other American surgeons had performed successful ovariectomies – Nathan Smith of Connecticut in 1821 and A.G. Smith, another Kentuckian, in 1823.

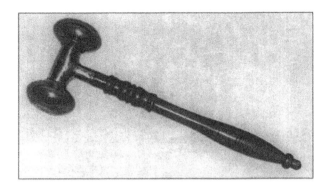

Figure 1.5 **The gavel used at the Royal College of Obstetricians and Gynaecologists, London; it is made from a piece of wood from Ephraim McDowell's home.**

The cynical reception of McDowell's first report is shown by an article in the *London Medical and Chirurgical Review* by Dr James Johnson, who wrote 'three cases of ovarian extirpation occurred, it would seem, some years ago in the practice of Dr McDowell of Kentucky, which were transmitted to the late John Bell and fell into the hands of Mr Lizars. We candidly confess that we are rather sceptical respecting these statements, and we are rather surprised that Mr Lizars himself should put implicit confidence in them'. However, the publication of McDowell's second report made even the unbelieving English repent, and in 1826 the same author wrote:

A back settlement of America – Kentucky – has beaten the mother country, nay, Europe itself, with all the boasted surgeons thereof, in the fearful and formidable operation of gastrotomy, with extraction of diseased ovaria....There were circumstances in the narrative of some of the first three cases that raised misgivings in our minds, for which uncharitableness we ask pardon of God and of Dr. McDowell of Danville. Two additional cases now published...are equally wonderful as those with which our readers are already acquainted.

Since that time the stature of McDowell in surgical history has grown (Figure 1.6). It is now acknowledged that he was the father not only of ovariotomy but also of abdominal surgery.

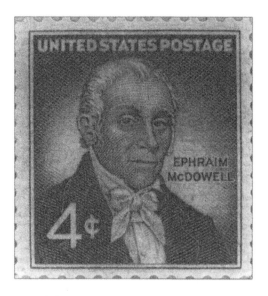

Figure 1.6 **Ephraim McDowell immortalised by the United States Postal Service.** (Courtesy of the Royal College of Obstetricians and Gynaecologists, London.)

What of Ephraim McDowell, the man? Physically, he was imposing, nearly six feet in height, erect, with the florid complexion of a countryman. His eyes were black, and their piercing lustre was often the subject of comment. He was physically strong, active, eschewed tobacco in any form, but occasionally took a nip of whisky or cherry bounce; he preferred the latter, which was whisky with macerated cherries, sugar and spices. His dress was neat and usually black. Although he had a creditable library, he was no writer, and the two reports on the ovarian surgery were his only contributions to the medical literature; would that any of us were privileged to make such contributions! He was comfortably off, had a farm, and, in the best Kentuckian tradition, bred fine horses. He married at the age of thirty-one; his bride was Miss Sarah Shelby, the eighteen-year-old daughter of the first governor of Kentucky. They had two sons and four daughters.

McDowell died in 1830, at fifty-nine years of age, after a two-week illness of 'an acute attack of inflammation of the stomach' – perhaps acute appendicitis. What a pity that abdominal surgery had not progressed a little further by then.

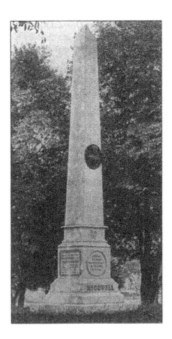

Figure 1.7 **Memorial at the burial place of Dr Ephraim McDowell and Mrs McDowell in Danville.** (Reprinted with permission from Schachner A. *Ephraim McDowell: Father of Ovariotomy and Founder of Abdominal Surgery.* Philadelphia, JR Lippincott 1921.)

McDowell was buried in the family burial ground some five miles from Danville, but in 1879 his remains were removed to what is now called McDowell Park, once the old Danville cemetery. The site is marked by a fine memorial shaft in Virginia granite erected by the Kentucky State Medical Society. The inscription reads, 'Beneath this shaft rests Ephraim McDowell, M.D., the father of ovariotomy, who by originating a great surgical operation became a benefactor of his race, known and honoured throughout the civilised world'. (Figure 1.7).

But what about the heroine of this story, Mrs Jane Todd Crawford? Fortunately, Dr Robert S. Sparkman of Baylor University Medical Centre has performed a valuable piece of historical research and in his Presidential Address to the Southern Surgical Association in 1978 gave a detailed account of her life. She was born in December 1763 and married Thomas Crawford when she was thirty years of age. The ceremony was performed by the Reverend Samuel

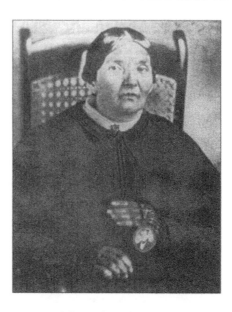

Figure 1.8 **Daguerreotype of Jane Todd Crawford taken in either 1840 or 1841, a year or so before her death at the age of 78.** (Reprinted with permission from Schachner A. *Ephraim McDowell: Father of Ovariotomy and Founder of Abdominal Surgery.* Philadelphia, JR Lippincott 1921.)

Houston, whose infant cousin, also named Sam, was later to become the hero of Tennessee and Texas.

In 1805, the Crawfords moved to Kentucky and erected their log cabin. In the very year of Mrs Crawford's operation (1809), only thirty-five miles away from the Crawford cabin in a similar log cabin, an infant named Abe Lincoln was born.

The year after Mrs Crawford's surgery, the Crawfords moved from Motley's Glen, Green County, first to northern Kentucky and then to Indiana, where Mr Crawford was a substantial landowner and a representative in the Indiana legislature. Mrs Crawford died in 1842 at the age of seventy-eight and was buried in Graysville, Indiana, where her gravestone is preserved and a modem bronze memorial tablet has been erected (Figure 1.8).

As a pleasant final note, in 1932, the Kentucky State Highway Department designated the road from Motley's Glen, Green County, to Danville the 'Jane Todd Crawford Trail'. How different now the journey is along this highway by car from Mrs Crawford's horseback ride across that frontier country in midwinter of 1809!

Bibliography

Price JA. The early ovariotomists – Pioneers in abdominal surgery. *Ulster Med J* 36:1, 1967.

Schachner A. *Ephraim MacDowell: Father of Ovariotomy and Founder of Abdominal Surgery*. Philadelphia, JL Lippincott, 1921.

Sparkman RS. The woman in the case. Jane Todd Crawford 1763–1842. *Ann Surg* 189:529, 1979.

Spencer HR. The history of ovariotomy. In *Sidelights on the History of Medicine*. Edited by Sir Zachary Cope, London, Butterworths, 1957, p. 188.

2

LIGATION OF THE ABDOMINAL AORTA

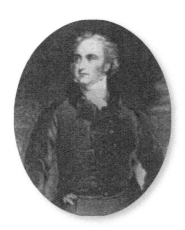

I can claim, without fear of contradiction, that Sir Astley Cooper (Figure 2.1) of Guy's Hospital, London, was the father of arterial surgery. I make this assertion not only on the evidence that he was a pioneer in the ligation of the common carotid and the external iliac arteries and, as we shall investigate here, the first to tie the abdominal aorta, but also on the fact that these surgical feats were backed by profound anatomical and physiological studies.

As a medical student, young Cooper carried out studies of the collateral circulation following ligation of the femoral and brachial arteries in dogs. His experimental work continued throughout his active professional life, and series of investigations were performed on the cerebral circulation in dogs. He showed that both carotid arteries could be tied without obvious harm, since the dog, with its comparatively small cerebrum, depended more on the vertebral

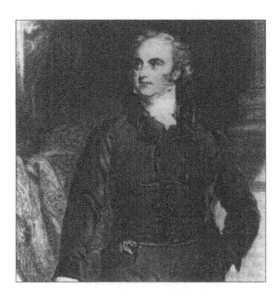

Figure 2.1 **Sir Astley Cooper.** (Courtesy of the Royal College of Surgeons of England, London.)

arteries than on the carotids. Indeed, ligation of both vertebral arteries was usually fatal, and compression of the vertebrals following ligation of both carotids rendered the dog unconscious. One dog actually survived serial ligation of both carotids and both vertebral arteries and lived for nine months as a pet before being killed to demonstrate the collateral circulation that had developed. Cooper finally demonstrated that a dog could survive ligation of the abdominal aorta, although there was some weakness of the lower limbs. It has been stated that Cooper was the first surgeon to ligate the carotid artery, but in fact, the credit for this goes to a naval surgeon, David Fleming, who tied the carotid artery in October 1803 for a secondary haemorrhage following a cut throat. This operation was carried out in the sick bay of His Majesty's Ship *Tennant,* a two-decker of eighty guns, cruising off the Spanish coast. The patient, Mark Jackson, a ship's servant, had almost exsanguinated but made an uninterrupted recovery following his emergency operation. We should be grateful indeed to Surgeon Commander J.J. Keevil for recording this vignette of naval surgical history.

Cooper's first case of carotid ligation was a forty-four-year-old woman named Mary Edwards. Cooper writes, 'The swelling occupied two-thirds of the right side of the neck, pulsated very strongly and the integument at the most prominent part of the tumour appeared very thin'. The operation was performed on November 1, 1805. A two-inch incision was made along the inner edge of the sternomastoid just above the clavicle. The common carotid artery was exposed, the vagus separated, and two thread ligatures passed around the vessel and firmly tied. All pulsation in the tumour immediately ceased. At first progress was good, but on the eighth day she developed a transient weakness of the left arm and leg. Although strength returned to the limbs, extensive inflammation occurred within the sac, and the patient died on November 21. An autopsy revealed that 'the cause of her death was the inflammation of aneurysmal sac and of the adjacent parts, by which the size of the tumour became so increased as to press on the pharynx and prevent deglutition, and upon the larynx, so as to excite coughing, and to impede respiration'.

A second opportunity came three years later when Humphrey Humphries, fifty years of age and a porter, was admitted with an aneurysm on the left side of the neck about the size of a walnut, extending from the angle of the jaw to the thyroid cartilage. On June 22, 1808, the carotid artery was tied and divided between the ligatures. On this occasion, recovery was uneventful, and the patient returned to his employment on September 14. He survived for thirteen years, died of a cerebral haemorrhage, and was subjected to a careful autopsy.

On the same afternoon on which he ligated Humphries' carotid, Cooper carried out ligation of the external iliac artery for a large femoral aneurysm – surely an operating list of which any modern vascular surgeon would be proud. The patient, a thirty-nine-year-old man, recovered. Cooper performed this operation on nine patients, two of them doctors; there was only one death, a secondary haemorrhage on the fifteenth day. The extraperitoneal approach to the external iliac artery bears Cooper's name to this day.

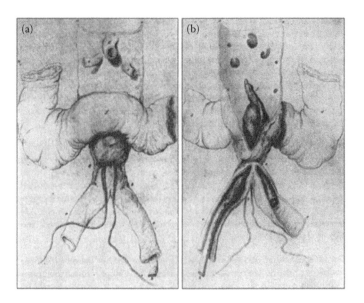

Figure 2.2 **Contemporary drawings of Sir Astley Cooper's specimen of ligation of the abdominal aorta. (a) Anterior view. (b) Posterior dissection.** (Reprinted with permission from *Guy's Hospital Reports*, 1940–1941.)

Undoubtedly Cooper's most famous vascular operation was ligature of the aorta (Figure 2.2), and we can do no better than to quote from his own description of the case:

> Charles Hutson, a porter aet. 38, was admitted into Guy's Hospital on the 9th April 1817, for an aneurysm in the left groin, situated partly above and partly below Poupart's ligament. On the third day after he had been in the hospital, the swelling increased to double its former size, and extended from three to four inches above Poupart's ligament to an equal distance below it and was of great magnitude...and the peritoneum was carried far from the lower part of the abdomen, in such a manner as to reach the common iliac artery, and to render an operation impracticable without opening the cavity of the peritoneum.
>
> He was occasionally bled, kept perfectly quiet, and pressure was applied on the tumour. June 19th, a slough was observed on the exterior part of the swelling below Poupart's ligament which, in part, separated on the 20th, and he had some bleeding

from the sac but it was easily stopped by a compress of lint, confined on the part by adhesive plaster. On the 22nd, after some slight exertion, he bled again but not profusely. [On the] 24th, the bleeding again recurred, but stopped spontaneously, [and on the] 25th, about half past 2 o'clock [he] bled profusely and became so much exhausted that his faeces passed off involuntarily; but Mr. Key, then my apprentice, succeeded in preventing immediate dissolution by pressure. At 9 o'clock the same evening I saw him, and found him in so reduced a state that he could not survive another haemorrhage, with which he was every moment threatened….As the only chance which remained of preventing his immediate dissolution by haemorrhage was by tying the aorta, I determined on doing it. The operation was performed as follows….

The patient's shoulders were slightly elevated by pillows, in order to relax as much as possible the abdominal muscles….1 then made an incision three inches long into the linea alba, giving it a slight curve to avoid the umbilicus. Having divided the linea alba, I made a small aperture into the peritoneum, and introduced my finger into the abdomen; and then with a probe-pointed bistoury enlarged the opening into the peritoneum to nearly the same extent as that of the external wound. During the progress of the operation, only one small convolution of intestine projected beyond the wound.

Having made a sufficient opening to admit my finger into the opening, I passed it between the intestines to the spine, and felt the aorta greatly enlarged, and beating with excessive force. By means of my finger nail, I scratched through the peritoneum on the left side of the aorta, and then gradually passed my finger between the aorta and the spine, and again penetrated the peritoneum, on the right side of the aorta.

I had now my finger under the artery, and by its side I conveyed the blunt aneurismal needle, armed with a single ligature behind it; and Mr. Key drew the ligature through the eye of the needle to the external wound, when the needle was withdrawn.

The next circumstance, which required considerable care, was the exclusion of the intestine from the ligature, the ends of which were brought together at the wound, and the finger was carried down between them, so as to remove every portion of the intestine from between the threads; the ligature was then tied, and its ends were left hanging out of the wound....The omentum was drawn behind the opening as far as the ligature would admit, so as to facilitate adhesion; and the edges of the wound were brought together by means of a quilled suture and adhesive plaster.

One of the students watching the operation, Edward Osler (uncle of Sir William Osler), who recorded the details in a letter, adds a dramatic touch in describing the climax. He writes that Cooper, looking around, said, 'Gentlemen, I have the pleasure of informing you that the aorta is now hooked upon my finger'.

At first all proceeded well. The normal right limb recovered its warmth and sensation, although the left limb, on the side of the aneurysm, was cold. The left leg became progressively more livid and cold, and the patient died forty hours after the operation.

At autopsy, Cooper's brilliant surgical skill was demonstrated: 'The thread had been passed around the aorta, about three-quarters of an inch above its bifurcation, and rather more than an inch below the part at which the duodenum crosses the artery; it had not included any portion of omentum, or intestine'.

The specimen has been preserved carefully to this day at St. Thomas's Hospital, London, and I am most grateful to my friend, Professor Sir Norman Browse, who provided me with a photograph of this unique preparation (Figure 2.3). One might say that the operation was one of mere surgical bravado, but this I would hotly deny. Cooper had already proved in his dog experiments (Figure 2.4) that there were sufficient collateral channels to maintain the blood supply to the lower limbs beyond the ligated aorta under normal circumstances, so the physiology of the operation was sound. Moreover, before performing the operation, Cooper had carefully worked out its surgical anatomy; when it became obvious that ligation of the aorta was indicated, Cooper

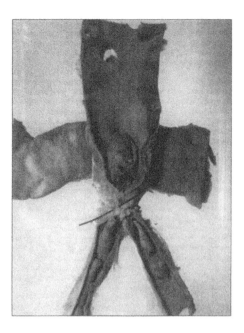

Figure 2.3 **The specimen of Sir Astley Cooper's ligation of the abdominal aorta as it is today, preserved in the Department of Surgery at St. Thomas's Hospital, London.** (Courtesy of Professor Sir Norman Browse.)

went to the post-mortem room, attempted to expose the aorta by a lateral retroperitoneal approach, found this to be impossible, and rehearsed a transperitoneal exposure. In his lecture notes, he ponders once more the possibility of a safer extraperitoneal exposure of the aorta: 'In an operation which I lately performed of tying the external iliac artery much above Poupart's ligament, I think I could with little difficulty have reached the aorta, by turning up the peritoneum without dividing it; and should I again wish to put a ligature on the aorta, I should prefer this method to the one I have before adopted'.

Obviously, with poor Charles Hutson, the case was late and neglected, with considerable disturbance of its collateral circulation and inevitable gangrene of the limb on the affected side. The fact that the opposite leg remained viable completely justified Cooper's hopes that survival could follow aortic ligation.

Unfortunately, Cooper never had the opportunity to repeat the operation. Indeed, although other surgeons followed his attempts,

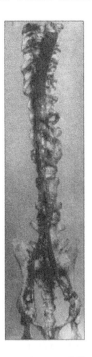

Figure 2.4 **Sir Astley Cooper's specimen of ligation of the aorta in the dog, injected to demonstrate its collateral circulation.** (Courtesy of Gordon Museum, Guy's Hospital, London.)

it remained for Rudolph Matas to report a successful ligation of the aorta for an aneurysm in 1925. The patient survived, only to die of pulmonary tuberculosis eighteen months later.

I must confess that Cooper is a particular hero of mine. Born in 1768, the son of a Norfolk country clergyman, he became an apprentice at the United Hospitals of Guy's and St. Thomas's, was appointed to the staff as surgeon to Guy's Hospital in 1800, where he spent the rest of his professional life. He served on the Council of the College of Surgeons from 1815 until his death in 1841 and was President in 1827 and again in 1836.

He was one of the hardest-working surgeons in history. At the height of his fame he was up every morning by six, often by five, and frequently by four. He would go straight to his dissecting room, where he would experiment until breakfast. From then until one o'clock he gave free consultations at his home. He then went to Guy's Hospital where he was met by up to 100 students who attended his rounds, his clinical lectures, and his operating sessions. Visits to private patients and operations in their homes would follow, then home by seven, a hurried meal, a ten-minute nap on the sofa, then out again to see more patients or to lecture; he never arrived home before midnight. Unfortunately, his married life was not a particular success, and he died without issue; certain things appear to be incompatible with retiring late and arising early.

His contributions to surgery were considerable. In addition to his work on arterial ligation, he was one of the first surgeons to carry out a successful disarticulation of the hip. This procedure was performed on January 15, 1824 on a soldier from the battle of Waterloo with chronic osteomyelitis of the femur following an above-knee amputation. A report on the operation appeared two days later in the *Lancet*. Cooper first ligated the femoral artery, then made an elliptical incision from below the inguinal ligament to about one-third along the back of the thigh, first dividing the skin and fascia and then the muscles. The head of the femur was disarticulated without difficulty. A total of four vessels were ligated and about twelve ounces of blood were lost. The skin flaps were brought together with a suture and strips of adhesive and a bandage put over the stump. The limb was removed in the space of twenty minutes, the securing of the blood vessels and the dressings occupied fifteen more; the whole operation was, therefore, completed in thirty-five minutes. During the operation the patient was extremely faint, but some wine being given him and some fresh air admitted, he recovered. The patient bore the operation with extraordinary fortitude and after all was finished, he said to Sir Astley 'that it was the hardest day's work he had ever gone through' to which Sir Astley replied 'that it was almost the hardest he ever had'.

Recovery was retarded by infection of the stump, which was relieved by loosening the dressings and strapping and by incision of an abscess. By March 19th the notes read 'Gains strength rapidly. Has been out of the ward twice during the past week and was each time wheeled about the squares of the hospital for a considerable period'. In August the patient was perfectly recovered and was living in the country residence of Sir Astley Cooper. It is an interesting light on Cooper's character that his interest in the welfare of his

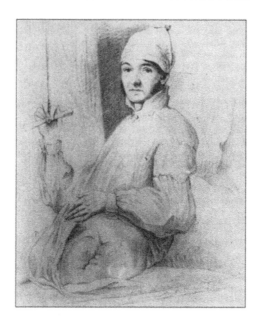

Figure 2.5 **Lithograph of Cooper's patient who underwent successful amputation through the hip joint.** (Reproduced by kind permission from Guy's Hospital Reports, 1939.)

patient extended so far as to provide convalescence for him in his own country house (Figure 2.5).

Astley Cooper also made major advances to our knowledge of the surgery of hernia, of the breast and of the management of fractures and dislocations. His most distinguished patient was George IV, whose sebaceous cyst of the scalp he removed. That famous operation merits a separate chapter later in this book.

Bibliography

Brock RC. *The Life and Work of Astley Cooper.* Edinburgh, ES Livingstone, 1952.

Cooper A. *The Lectures on the Principles and Practice of Surgery with Additional Notes and Cases by Frederick Tyrrell*, Vol 2. London, Thomas & George Underwood, 1824.

Eckhoff NL. An account of Sir Astley Cooper's first case of amputation at the hip joint, 16th January 1824. *Guys Hospital Reports* 98:9, 1939.

Keevil JJ. David Fleming and the operation for ligation of the carotid artery. *Br J Surg* 37:92, 1949.

Symonds CJ. Astley Paston Cooper. *Guy's Hospital Reports* 90:73, 1940.

3

RUPTURED ECTOPIC PREGNANCY

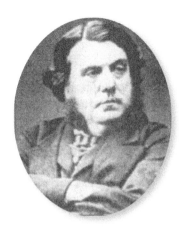

Only a little more than a century ago a ruptured ectopic pregnancy was a death sentence. In his book on extrauterine pregnancy published in 1876, John Parry wrote, 'Here is an accident which may happen to any wife in the most useful period of her existence, which good authorities have said is never cured; and for which, even in this age when science and art boast of such high attainments, no remedy either medical or surgical has been tried with a single success'. When we read that eminent authorities were advising the use of electric shocks, the injection of narcotic materials into the sac, and copious and frequent bleeding, one is hardly surprised at the rate of failure. Parry himself went on to suggest that the only remedy would be to open the abdomen and either to tie the bleeding vessels or to remove the sac entirely.

The first surgeon to perform a successful operation of the kind recommended by Parry was Robert Lawson Tait (Figure 3.1) of Birmingham, England, and it is interesting that the suggestion that

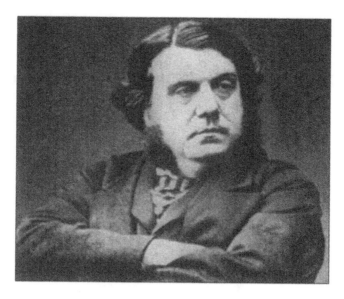

Figure 3.1 **Robert Lawson Tait.** (Courtesy of the Wellcome Institute for the History of Medicine, London.)

he should operate came from a general practitioner. The dramatic story involves three successive cases described vividly in Tait's own words:

> In the summer of 1881 I was asked by Mr. Hallwright to see with him in consultation a patient who had arrived by train from London in a condition of serious illness diagnosed by Mr. Hallwright as probably haemorrhage into the peritoneal cavity from a ruptured tubal pregnancy. The patient was blanched and collapsed, the uterus was fixed by a doughy mass in the pelvis and there was clearly a considerable amount of effusion in the peritoneum. I agreed with Mr. Hallwright as to the nature of the lesion. This gentleman made the bold suggestion that I should open the abdomen and remove the ruptured tube. The suggestion staggered me and I am ashamed to say that I did not receive it favourably....I declined to act on Mr. Hallwright's request and a further haemorrhage killed the patient. A post mortem examination revealed the perfect accuracy of the diagnosis. I carefully inspected the

specimen which was removed and I found that if I had tied the broad ligament and removed the ruptured tube I should have completely arrested the haemorrhage and I now believe that had I done this the patient's life would have been saved.

The second opportunity came eighteen months later, in the summer of 1883, when Tait was consulted by Mr Spackman of nearby Wolverhampton with a similar case. The patient was clearly dying, but Tait operated; it was the first occasion when an active surgical attempt was made to save a life under such circumstances. As Tait records, 'We got her to bed alive and that is all that can be said....I thought very much about this case for it was a bitter disappointment. I thought I should achieve a triumph and I had only a failure'. He resolved then that in any future case he would ignore the bleeding, go for the source of the haemorrhage, the broad ligament, tie it at its base and then remove debris and clots at leisure. The next patient presented herself on March 1, 1883. Tait was consulted by Dr Page of Solihull, a suburb of Birmingham, with a patient who had a fixed mass in the pelvis and whose menstruation had been arrested for about three months. She had a high pulse, an elevated temperature, and was in great pain. Tait writes:

> I advised abdominal section and found the abdomen full of clot. The right fallopian tube was ruptured and from it a placenta was protruding. I tied the tube and removed it. I searched for, but could not find, the foetus and I suppose it got lost among the folds of intestine and there was absorbed.... The patient made a very protracted convalescence but she is now perfectly well.
>
> Within a year Tait had operated on three additional patients, and four years later, in 1888, he was able to report thirty-nine cases with only two deaths, including his first attempt.

Tait, a remarkable man, was one of the fathers of abdominal surgery. Indeed, one medical historian went so far as to say that the three dominating figures of nineteenth century surgery were Joseph Lister, James Simpson and Robert Lawson Tait. Tait was born in Edinburgh on May 1, 1845. His father was a vintner, and his mother an irascible lady from whom he no doubt inherited his irritability and temper. He was a pupil of the great Sir James Young Simpson, Professor of Obstetrics in Edinburgh, who introduced chloroform into midwifery and surgery in 1847. Tait bore a striking resemblance to his professor, and indeed there were rumours that he was Simpson's natural son. Apart from the resemblance there seems to be little evidence to support this gossip, which secretly amused Tait.

He qualified in 1866, moved to Birmingham at twenty-five years of age, and spent the rest of his active life there until his death from uraemia due to renal stones at the early age of fifty-four in 1899 (Figures 3.2 and 3.3). Apart from his work on ectopic pregnancy, Tait pioneered the surgery of ovarian cysts and tumours, closely

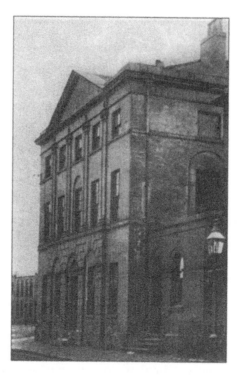

Figure 3.2 **No. 8 The Crescent, Birmingham. Site of the Women's Hospital from 1871 to 1878. Lawson Tait's private nursing home from 1882 to 1889.** (Courtesy of Professor Sir Geoffrey Slaney.)

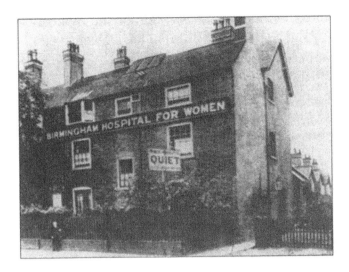

Figure 3.3 **The Women's Hospital, Birmingham (1878–1905) – the scene of much of Lawson Tait's surgery.** (Courtesy of Professor Sir Geoffrey Slaney.)

following on the early work of Spencer Wells in this field. His surgical skill is shown by the publication in 1886 of 137 consecutive cases of ovariotomy performed without a death. In 1879, he carried out the first cholecystotomy performed in Europe – the second ever performed in the world – in which he removed a large stone impacted at the neck of the gallbladder. Within five years he was able to report thirteen more cases with only one death. In 1880, he was the first to diagnose and successfully remove an acutely inflamed appendix.

He was a short, stout man with a magnificent head, a thick bull neck, corpulent body, pudgy legs, and small hands and feet; he was described as having the body of Bacchus and the head of Jove. His voice could be soft and musical; he would sing sweetly and yet, when in rage, would roar like a lion. Many observers commented on his marvellous rapidity and dexterity as a surgeon. His technique was simplicity itself. He operated in small nursing homes with the patient laid on a plain wooden table. He would remove his jacket, roll up his sleeves, and scrupulously prepare his hands with soap and water. The patient's abdomen would be carefully cleansed, first with turpentine and then with soap and water, and his instruments were sterilised by boding; he was one of the pioneers of aseptic rather than antiseptic surgery, and indeed he attacked Listerism as not only unnecessary but dangerous.

The contributions of this surgeon are best summed up by William Mayo who said, 'The cavities of the body were a sealed book until the father of modern abdominal surgery, Lawson Tait, carried the sense of sight into the abdominal cavity'.

Bibliography

McKay WIS. *Lawson Tait – His Life and Work.* London, Ballière, Tindall, and Cox, 1922.

Shepherd JA. *Lawson Tait – The Rebellious Surgeon, 1848–1899.* Kansas, Coronado Press, 1980.

4

THE FIRST SUCCESSFUL GASTRECTOMY

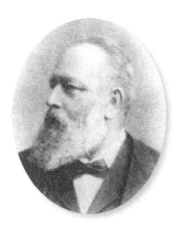

Today gastrectomy is a routine surgical procedure that any competent surgeon anywhere in the world is expected to perform efficiently, neatly, and well and with, in a reasonably fit patient, a good ninety-five percent chance of a speedy and safe recovery. It is perhaps worth remembering that this operation is just over a century old.

In April 1879, Jules Pean (Figure 4.1) of Paris performed a resection of a pyloric cancer in a cachectic patient who died on the fifth postoperative day. In November 1880, Ludwig Rydigier (Figure 4.2) of Culm, Poland, attempted the second gastrectomy in history, but his patient also died of exhaustion only twelve hours postoperatively. Meantime, in Vienna, at the great Surgical University Clinic of the Allgemeine Krankenhaus, Theodor Billroth (Figure 4.3) was keeping his assistants busy in the laboratory studying the technique of gastric resection in the dog. They were

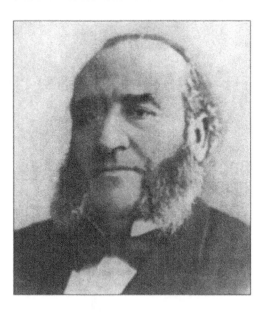

Figure 4.1 **Jules Péan (1830–1898). First surgeon to perform a gastrectomy, but with a fatal outcome.** (Reprinted with permission from Meade RH. *An Introduction to the History of General Surgery.* Philadelphia, WB Saunders, 1968, 204.)

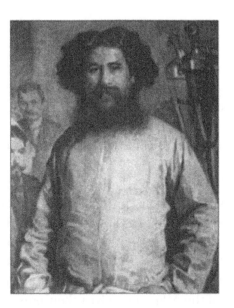

Figure 4.2 **Ludwig Rydigier (1850–1920).** (Photograph taken by H.E. of the portrait in the Surgical Clinic, Nicholaus Copernicus Academy of Medicine, Cracow.)

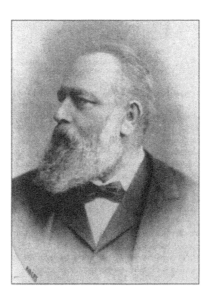

Figure 4.3 **Theodor Billroth (1829–1894).** (Courtesy of the Royal College of Surgeons of England, London.)

able to demonstrate that survival was undoubtedly possible and eliminated the question of whether the gastric juice would dissolve the scar tissue in the healing anastomosis.

In January 1881, one of Billroth's favourite assistants, Anton Wölfler (Figure 4.4), a thirty-year-old Czechoslovakian, called his chief to see a forty-three year-old woman, Thérèse Heller, who had all the symptoms of a malignant pyloric obstruction. Her symptoms dated back to October of the previous year; she was now bedridden and extremely wasted with a thin, rapid pulse, continuous vomiting, and a palpable tumour in the epigastrium. At this stage, she was able to retain only small amounts of sour milk. The poor woman was obviously close to death.

Billroth had planned the operation in great detail. Preparations consisted of washing out the stomach with fourteen litres of lukewarm water and administering peptone enemas. On January 29, 1881, the historic operation was performed. One of the private assistants administered chloroform, and an antiseptic technique was used. Wölfler assisted, and the operating room was heated to twenty degrees centigrade. A transverse incision was made over the

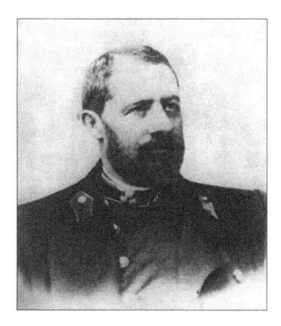

Figure 4.4 **Anton Wölfler (1850–1917).** (Reprinted with permission from Herwitz A, Degenshein GA. *Milestones in Modern Surgery.* Philadelphia, Harper and Row, 1958.)

tumour which, under the anaesthetic, was found to be movable and the size of a medium apple.

It took only a few minutes to expose the mass through the wasted abdominal wall; it proved to be an unpleasant nodular infiltrating carcinoma of the pylorus, involving more than one-third of the lower portion of the stomach. Its size made it difficult to deliver, and care was taken by Billroth to ligate the blood vessels along the greater and lesser borders of the stomach. A great anxiety was whether or not the stump of the stomach would pull over sufficiently to reach the duodenum, but, the healthy tissues having been divided about one inch on the stomach side of the growth, the cut ends could indeed be brought together. The oblique wound in the stomach was sutured from below upwards until the opening was just big enough to fit the duodenum, altogether some fifty sutures of silk were employed. The whole area was mopped out with a two per cent carbolic lotion, and the abdominal wound was then closed. The operation (Figure 4.5) lasted one and a half hours, including

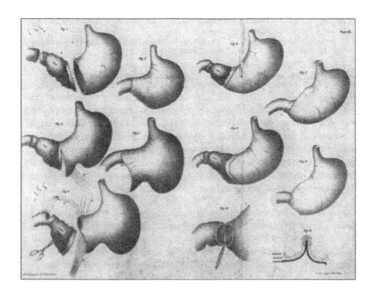

Figure 4.5 **Operative procedure on Frau Heller.** (Reprinted with permission from Billroth T. *Clinical Surgery. Extracts from the Reports of Surgical Practice between the Years 1860–1876.* London, The New Sydenham Society, 1891.)

the slow induction of anaesthetic. I am a talkative surgeon myself, and I was particularly interested to read that the whole time passed in complete silence!

Much to everyone's delight there was no weakness, vomiting, or pain after the operation. In the first twenty-four hours only ice was allowed by mouth, but the following day teaspoons of sour milk were given. There was a little pain that was easily relieved with small injections of morphine. By the end of the week the patient's condition was excellent. The wound was healing well, and the patient was moved to a room in the general ward so that she could chat with the other patients.

The excised specimen (Figure 4.6) showed an extensive cancer that had so narrowed the pylorus that it could just admit the shaft of a feather. This brave lady died of diffuse metastases in the liver and omentum only four months later, yet her courage in submitting herself to an operation, which was just as great a step into the unknown as the first fiver or heart transplantations, laid the foundations of modern abdominal surgery. By 1890, Billroth

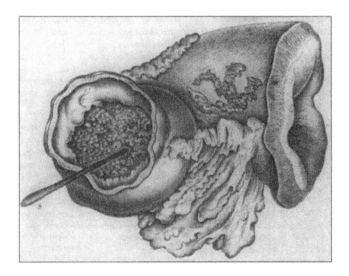

Figure 4.6 **Resected specimen of stomach of Frau Heller. Note that only a fine probe can be passed through the obstructing tumour.** (Reprinted with permission from Billroth T. Clinical Surgery. Extracts from the Reports of Surgical Practice between the Years 1860–1876. London, The New Sydenham Society, 1891.)

and his team had performed forty-one gastric resections for cancer with nineteen successes.

Billroth was undoubtedly one of the surgical giants of all time. He was born in April 1829, of Swedish parents on the island of Rugen, which is now in East Germany. His father was the local pastor. He graduated from the University of Berlin and became an assistant to the great Bernhard von Langenbeck. In 1860, at the age of thirty-one he became Professor of Surgery at Zurich, where he remained for seven years, until he was appointed by the Emperor Franz Joseph to the Chair of Surgery in Vienna. He was a pioneer in experimental surgery, a daring operator and an inspiring teacher. In 1871, he showed that oesophagectomy was possible in the dog, and in 1872 he performed the first total laryngectomy. He pioneered the hindquarter amputation, excision of bladder cancer and tumours of the bowel, and between his first successful gastrectomy in 1881 and his death in 1894, he personally carried out thirty-four resections of the stomach for cancer. Billroth was the founder of the modern concept of reporting the total clinical experience of a department, and his reports from Vienna, fortunately available in English translation, make fascinating reading. They include operative mortality, complications, and the five-year follow-up so dear to the surgeon of today. He sounded a warning note, however: 'Statistics', he wrote, 'are like women; mirrors of purest virtue and truth, or like whores, to use as one pleases'.

As a teacher he, more than any other, was responsible for the great German school of surgery, and his pupils included Johann von Mikulicz, who became Professor of Surgery in Breslau; Carl Gussenbauer, who succeeded him to the Chair of Surgery in Vienna; Vincenz Czerny, who obtained the Chair of Surgery in Heidelberg; Wölfler, who in the same year as the first successful gastrectomy performed the first gastroenterostomy with survival; and Anton von Eiselberg, who became Professor of the First Surgical Service in Vienna and who, in turn, trained nineteen surgical chiefs. In the midst of all this professional activity, Billroth found time to be an accomplished musician – he was an intimate friend of Johannes Brahms – and to play a prominent part in Austrian politics as a member of the Upper House of Parliament. A master among men, he well deserves to be remembered eponymously each time we use the term 'Billroth I gastrectomy'.

Bibliography

Billroth T. *Clinical Surgery. Extracts from the Reports of Surgical Practice between the Years 1860–1876* (Translated from the original by CT Dent). London, New Sydenham Society, 1891.

Rutledge RH: In commemoration of Theodor Billroth on the 150th anniversary of his birth. *Surg Gynecol Obstet* 86:672–693, 1979.

5

SPLENECTOMY FOR RUPTURE
OF THE SPLEEN

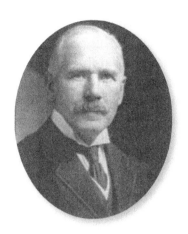

The years between 1870 and 1900 saw a burgeoning of surgery for the treatment of acute abdominal emergencies throughout the Western world such as had never been seen before and which is unlikely ever to happen again. The reasons for this are several. First, the introduction of ether anaesthesia by Morton in 1846 (*see Chapter 8*) and of chloroform by J.Y. Simpson of Edinburgh the following year abolished the agonies of the surgical knife and made it possible to operate upon the abdomen. Second, Lister's introduction of antiseptic surgery, commencing in 1867 (*see Chapter 9*) and the development of aseptic surgery, particularly by the German school, made abdominal surgery now not only possible but reasonably safe. Finally, surgeons were able to observe pathology in the operating theatre, which Moynihan termed 'the pathology of the living', so that a new understanding of many hitherto mysterious phenomena now became better understood.

For example, the mythical 'perityphlitis' was replaced by the true pathology of acute appendicitis.

One by one, the acute abdominal emergencies that had hitherto been almost invariably fatal were shown to be amenable to surgical cure. In 1871, Jonathan Hutchinson of the London Hospital operated on a female child aged two years with intestinal obstruction due to an intussusception, which was actually prolapsing from the anus. Up to that time, this condition was almost invariably fatal except in those rare cases where sloughing of the intussusceptum had occurred. Under chloroform, Hutchinson opened the abdomen through a lower mid-line incision, easily reduced the six-inch long mass and the child made a good recovery from this three-minute operation. Lawson Tait of Birmingham performed the first successful salpingectomy for ruptured ectopic pregnancy in 1883 (*see Chapter 3*). It was Tait also who carried out the first successful appendicectomy in 1880. He removed a gangrenous appendix and invaginated the stump. Unfortunately he failed to publish this case until 1890, by which time others had reported successful operations. Hale in New York in 1886 reported the first successful operation, although in his case the gangrenous appendix was found in an irreducible inguinal hernia. In 1887, T.G. Morton in Philadelphia correctly diagnosed appendicular disease, opened an abscess and removed the appendix with good recovery of his patient. The first successful repair of a perforated gastric ulcer was performed by Heusner in Wuppertal, Germany in 1892. He operated on a man aged forty-one in his own home by candle-light. Recovery was stormy, complicated by a left-sided empyema, which required drainage, but there was eventual recovery. The first successful repair in England was performed by Hastings Gilford of Reading the following year.

The spleen is the commonest viscus to be damaged in closed abdominal injuries, particularly a severe crushing blow to the left lower chest or abdomen; the commonest cause of this today is a road traffic accident. Although spontaneous healing may occasionally occur, untreated and without surgical treatment the majority of patients with this injury will die of exsanguination. Rather surprisingly, therefore, there seemed to be diffidence by surgeons

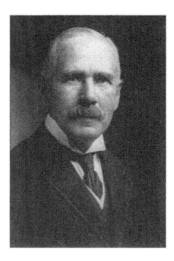

Figure 5.1 **Sir William Arbuthnot Lane.** (Courtesy of the Royal College of Surgeons of England, London.)

to open the abdomen in this condition during the pioneer days of abdominal surgery and to remove the ruptured spleen. Indeed, first attempts at splenectomy for closed injury appear not to have been made until the last decade of the nineteenth century. The first two unsuccessful attempts to be recorded were reported by Sir William Arbuthnot Lane (Figure 5.1) of Guy's Hospital, London who briefly described two cases in the *Lancet* of 1892. The first was a boy of fifteen who fell off a brougham, landed on its pole and was operated on by Lane shortly afterwards. A pulped spleen was removed, but the patient lived only five hours. The second was a boy of four who received a blow on the abdomen from the pole of a carriage. The spleen was completely ruptured, splenectomy was performed but, again, the child survived only a few hours. The following year, Friedrich Trendelenburg, Professor of Surgery in Leipzig, reported a further case of unsuccessful splenectomy for closed trauma and indeed published further fatal cases in 1896 and 1898.

It fell to Riegner, Chief Surgeon at the All Saints Hospital in Breslau, to have the distinction of performing the first successful splenectomy for closed splenic trauma on May 18, 1893. The patient was a fourteen-year-old labourer who fell two floors from scaffolding, striking his abdomen on a board. He was observed in hospital and by next morning he was increasingly pale with a pulse of 120. The abdomen was distended, painful and dull in the left flank. When finally the pulse reached 140, operation was decided upon. The abdomen was opened through a large mid-line incision. Immediately about 1.5 litres of blood poured out. At first, it was thought it was coming from the region of the liver and a long diagonal incision was made below the right costal margin. However, no injury to the liver was found. The intestines were then taken from the abdominal cavity and packed in warm saline compresses. It was then noted that particles of spleen could be seen in the masses of blood clot on the left side of the abdomen. A diagonal incision was therefore made on the left side and the spleen was seen to be completely severed in its middle. The lower half was lying free in the abdomen and removed. The splenic vessels were tied and the upper half of the spleen excised. All the abdominal incisions were closed with simple sutures; resuscitation comprised 300gr of normal saline infused subcutaneously into each of the arms and thighs. The boy's recovery was complicated by gangrene of the left foot, which required a through-knee amputation, but he recovered and was sent home with an artificial limb on October 17.

It was not until September 11, 1895 that Sir Charles Alfred Ballance (Figure 5.2) carried out the second successful splenectomy for closed trauma. This was on a schoolboy aged ten who had been struck by a cricket ball on the left side of the abdomen five days before admission (Figure 5.3). This patient, and two other cases, a woman run over by a hansom cab and a man of thirty-six who had fallen across an iron girder, were reported in great detail at the Clinical Society of London by Ballance together with his assistant, Bernard Pitts. A further successful case from St Thomas's was reported by Ballance in 1898 in a boy of fourteen who fell out of a tree.

Charles Ballance (1856–1936) was a student at St Thomas's Hospital, London. He gained a gold medal in surgery in his final examination and another gold medal for his Master of Surgery degree. He was appointed aural surgeon at St Thomas's Hospital, where he made important contributions to the surgery of the

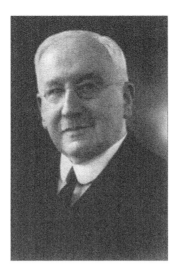

Figure 5.2 **Sir Charles Alfred Ballance.** (Courtesy of the Royal College of Surgeons of England, London.)

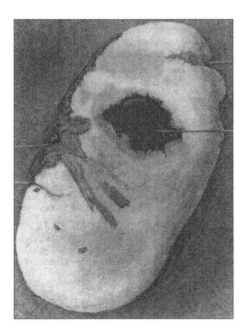

Figure 5.3 **Rupture of spleen from a cricket ball – Ballance's first successful splenectomy for trauma.** (Transactions of the Clinical Society, 1896. 29; 77–104.)

mastoid. He also served on the staff of the National Hospital for Nervous Diseases. He served as consultant surgeon during the First World War and was Vice President of the Council of the Royal College of Surgeons of England. Ballance spent much of his life involved in experimental surgery, being particularly interested in the parasitic theory of cancer, in tissue repair and, above all, in degeneration and regeneration of peripheral nerves. He described the shifting dullness in the right flank and fixed dullness in the left, which he claimed occurred in haemorrhage from the spleen. This, rather doubtful, physical sign is often referred to as 'Ballance's Sign'. I, personally, have never elicited it.

Bibliography

Cope Z. *A History of the Acute Abdomen*. London, Oxford University Press, 1965.

Ellis H. Jonathan Hutchinson (1829–1913). *J Med Biogr* 1:16, 1993.

Pitts B and Ballance CA. Three cases of splenectomy for rupture. *Trans the Clin Soc* 29:77, 1896.

Reigner O. Ein Fall von Milzextirpation nach traumatische Zerreisen. *Berliner Klinische Wochenschrift* 8:177, 1893.

6

RENAL TRANSPLANTATION

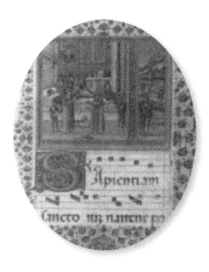

The story of the first successful homograft you may or may not believe. Cosmos and Damian were twin Christian physicians in Syria in the third century AD, who worked among the poor without fee. The Roman governor commanded the brothers to worship the pagan gods, and when they refused he ordered them both beheaded.

No sooner were they buried than there were reports of miraculous cures at the tomb at Cyrus. Two centuries later Justinian I, having himself benefited from visiting the grave, dedicated a temple to the twins at Constantinople and had their remains brought there from Syria. By the sixth century, the bones were removed to Rome, and the brothers became patron saints of medicine.

The story goes that a man afflicted with cancer of the leg spent the night in the church of St. Cosmos and St. Damian, where the two brothers appeared to him in a dream. One removed the

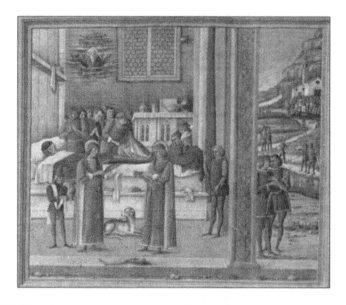

Figure 6.1 **The brothers Cosmos and Damian. The operation has been completed and the Moor's leg successfully grafted. Far in the background on the right, the crowd inspects the Moor's body. The original painting is a miniature in a fifteenth-century choir book now in the possession of the Society of Antiquaries in London; it has been attributed to both Andrea Mantegna and Guido da Ferrara.** (Courtesy of the Society of Antiquaries of London.)

diseased leg, while the other went to the cemetery of St. Peter in Chains, where he amputated the leg of a blackamoor who had died that very day and grafted it successfully onto the amputation stump (Figure 6.1). When the patient awoke the next morning, he found that his diseased leg had been replaced by a healthy black one. When disbelievers went to the grave of the donor and opened it, they found indeed the cancerous leg beside the body. This story has inspired artists from all over the world, and at least 1500 paintings of this miracle have been counted.

Organ homotransplantation, without saintly intervention, has had to wait until just a few years ago for similar success. The accumulation of knowledge concerning transplantation was slow. At the end of the eighteenth century, John Hunter transplanted teeth from one person to another with success, and also demonstrated that a human tooth could be transplanted to a cock's comb, teeth apparently being relatively inert antigenically. In 1804, Giuseppi Baronio demonstrated that free skin autografts in the sheep would survive; this is the experimental basis of much of modern plastic surgery. In the early twentieth century, Alexis Carrel, the pioneer of the vascular suture, carried out renal transplantations in dogs. He was clearly aware that although he could overcome the technical surgical problems, he was defeated by the biology of transplantation. In a letter to Theodor Kocher in 1914 he wrote, 'Concerning homoplastic transplantation (from one animal into another) of organs such as the kidney, I have never found positive results to continue after a few months, whereas in autoplastic transplantation the result was always positive. The biological side of the question has to be investigated very much more, and we must find out by what means to prevent the reaction of the organism against a new organ'.

The classical studies on skin grafting by Peter Medawar and his group during the Second World War clearly demonstrated that the rejection of a foreign tissue graft was an immunological mechanism. That skin grafts could be accepted between identical twins laid the basis for the exciting possibility that a sick identical twin might accept an organ graft from a healthy sibling.

Today, transplantation is accepted as a more or less routine procedure. Indeed, controversy seems to centre more on the shortage of donors and on the cost-effectiveness and the ethics of dialysis and transplantation programmes. Yet, to many of us, the very fact that organ transplantation has been achieved at all still seems quite amazing, and, indeed, the first successful kidney graft between identical twins was performed on December 23, 1954. This landmark in surgical achievement was reported thirteen months later in the *Journal of the American Medical Association* by John Merrill, Joseph Murray, Hartwell Harrison and Warren Guild from the medical and surgical services of the Peter Bent Brigham Hospital in Boston.

The patient was a twenty-four-year-old single man who presented with oedema and hypertension. His condition deteriorated over a five-month period, with the development of anaemia, vomiting, headaches and eventually convulsions. Since the patient had a twin brother, the possibility of homotransplantation of a kidney was considered, and he was transferred to the Peter Bent Brigham Hospital in October 1954.

On admission, the patient was thin, pale, drowsy and extremely disorientated. He had proteinuria, an Escherichia coli infection of the urine, and a blood urea nitrogen of 185 mg/dl. The haemoglobin was 6.7 g/dl. The patient was restless, was unable to tolerate oral feedings and became frankly psychotic. On the fourth hospital day he was treated by dialysis with the artificial kidney for a four-hour period. The response was good; he became mentally normal and was able to take food by mouth.

A full-thickness skin graft was exchanged between the twins, and a perfect take was obtained. The patient's condition continued to deteriorate, and by December 12 he was in congestive cardiac failure, with an enlarged liver, oedema of the legs up to the knees, a right-sided pleural effusion, papilloedema and a blood pressure of 220/146 mm Hg.

On December 16, thirty-one days after the original skin transplant, a biopsy was taken, and the graft appeared to have survived as normal skin. Because of this evidence of tissue compatibility, the twins were thought to be monozygotic. In addition, the twins' blood was found to be identical for all the eight blood-group systems then known. The hospital record of their birth showed that there was a common placenta, and moreover both twins had the relatively rare Darwin's tubercle of the ears, which their two siblings had not. The twins had identical eye colours, including iris structure and pigment patterns, which were markedly different from those of their siblings.

The crucial nephrectomy was carried out on December 23, 1954. Procedures were performed simultaneously on the donor and the recipient in adjacent operating rooms. A normal left kidney was removed from the healthy twin and grafted into the right iliac fossa of the patient in the extraperitoneal area (Figure 6.2). The donor renal artery was anastomosed to the internal iliac artery of the patient, the renal vein joined to the side of the common iliac vein, and the ureter implanted into the bladder; this technique has

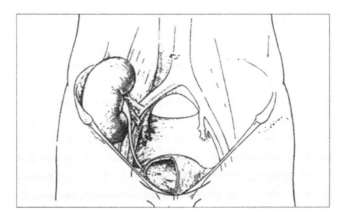

Figure 6.2 **Diagram of the first successful renal, graft. The renal artery is anastomosed end-to-end with the internal iliac, the renal vein end-to-side with the common iliac, and the ureter mucosa-to-mucosa with the bladder. This has served as the prototype for the technique of renal transplantations to this day.** (Reprinted with permission from Merrill JP. et al. *JAMA* 160:277, 1956.)

become the standard pattern in all renal transplants. The total operating time was three and a half hours. The total ischaemia of the donor kidney was one hour and twenty-two minutes. The entire kidney became turgid and pink immediately on release of the arterial clamps, and clear urine flowed copiously from the donor kidney.

The post-operative course was smooth, with primary healing of the wound, and the patient was discharged from the hospital on the thirty-seventh post-operative day. His twin brother also had an uneventful recovery and was allowed to return home after two weeks.

Subsequently, the patient had both of his diseased kidneys removed; they were shrunken and fibrosed and showed the appearances of diffuse, advanced chronic glomerulonephritis. Following this, the patient's blood pressure stabilised at almost normal levels and his urinary infection cleared. A year after the transplantation the patient was well, normotensive, and carrying on unlimited activity without apparent physical disability. Intravenous urography showed prompt excretion of dye in good concentration, although the ureter appeared somewhat dilated and tortuous.

Surely, if any operation is to receive that much-worn accolade, 'a major breakthrough', this was it. By 1961, at least twenty-five more renal transplantations had taken place between human identical twins; of these, the Boston team performed seventeen. Three of their patients died, one from thrombosis of the renal vessels and two from glomerulonephritis of the transplant in patients who had suffered from it before surgery. Of the remaining patients, the longest survivor was alive seven years after surgery.

There still remained, of course, the tremendous problems of the immunological barrier to transplantation. In 1959, R.S. Schwartz and W. Dameshek showed that the treatment of rabbits with 6-mercaptopurine produced a long-lasting immunological tolerance to human serum albumin. After seeing this report, a young English surgical registrar at St. Mary's Hospital, London, Roy Calne, decided to investigate the action of 6-mercaptopurine on renal homografts in dogs. This work was carried out at the Harvard Medical School with a Harkness Research Fellowship. His demonstration that the experimental animal could accept a completely unmatched kidney graft from another donor using this purine analogue provided the basis on which subsequent human transplantation of donor organs has depended. Calne is now Emeritus Professor of Surgery at the University of Cambridge, where his unit has become a Mecca to surgeons and research workers in this field. He has not only been knighted, but is one of the few surgeons to have been elected a Fellow of the Royal Society. Among my happiest memories is the fact that Calne was my second in command at Westminster Hospital Medical School after the surgical unit was founded in 1962, and it was there that he carried out his first thirteen human renal transplantations.

Bibliography

Calne RY. *Renal Transplantation*. London, Edward Arnold, 1963.

Calne RY. *Art, Surgery and Transplantation*. London, Williams & Wilkins, 1996.

Malinin TI. *Surgery and Life. The Extraordinary Career of Alexis Correl*. New York, Harcourt Brace Jovanovich, 1979.

Merrill JP, Murray JE, Harrison JH et al. Successful homotransplantation of the human kidney between identical twins. *JAMA* 160:271, 1956.

Part II

INNOVATIONS

7

I DRESSED THE WOUND AND
GOD HEALED HIM

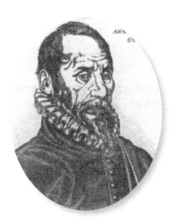

Every time an orthopaedic surgeon deals with a traumatised limb, he should utter a silent prayer to a sixteenth-century French surgeon, a particular hero of mine, Ambroise Paré (Figure 7.1).

Among his many contributions, Paré did two great services for surgery and therefore for suffering mankind; first, he showed that wounds need not be cauterised with boiling oil, and second, he replaced the red-hot iron with the ligature in controlling the bleeding from great vessels during amputations. By these two discoveries, both based on close clinical observation and immense experience, he saved thousands of wounded soldiers from the tortures previously inflicted on them.

Paré was born in the little town of Laval, France, in 1510, the son of a barber. At twenty-two years of age, he came to Paris as an apprentice to a barber-surgeon and later moved to the great

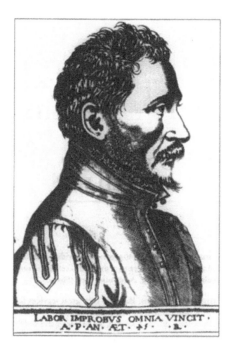

Figure 7.1 **Ambroise Paré at forty-five years of age. Engraving attributed to Jean le Royer, 1561.** (Reprinted with permission from Keynes G. *The Apologie and Treatise of Ambroise Paré.* New York, Dover Publications, 1951.)

Hotel Dieu as compagnon-chirurgeon, which I suppose we could translate as a resident. In that immense medieval hospital, he gained great experience.

Perhaps because he could not afford to pay the fees for admission to the ranks of the barber-surgeon, Paré, at twenty-six years of age, started his career as a military surgeon. In those days, there was no organised medical care for the humble private soldiers of armies in the field. Surgeons were attached to individual generals and other important personages, and might, if they wished, give what aid they could to the common soldiers in their spare time. Otherwise, the soldiers had to rely on the rough help of their companions or of a motley crowd of horse-doctors, farriers, quacks and mountebanks. Paré was appointed surgeon to the Duke of Montejan, who was Colonel-General of the French infantry. This, his first of many campaigns, took him to Turin, and it was here in 1537 that he made the fundamental observations he described so brilliantly in his magnificent book, *The Apologie and Treatise.*

> I was at that time a fresh-water surgeon, since I had not yet seen treated wounds made by firearms. It is true I had read in Jean de Vigo in his first book of 'Wounds in General' chapter 8, that wounds made by firearms are poisoned because of the powder. For their cure he advised their cauterisation with oil of elders mixed with a little theriac. To not fail, this oil must be applied boiling, even though this would cause the wounded extreme pain. I wished to know first how to apply it, how the other surgeons did their first dressings, which was to apply the oil as boiling as possible. So I took heart to do as they did. Finally, my oil was exhausted and I was forced instead to apply a digestive made of egg yolk, rose oil and turpentine. That night I could not sleep easily, thinking that by failure of cauterising, I would find the wounded in whom I had failed to put the oil dead of poisoning. This made me get up early in the morning to visit them. There, beyond my hope, I found those on whom I had used the digestive medication feeling little pain in their wounds, without inflammation and swelling, having rested well through the night. The others on whom I had used the oil I found feverish, with great pain, swelling and inflammation around their wounds. Then I resolved never again to so cruelly burn the poor wounded by gunshot.

What a wonderful description of one of the earliest controlled experiments! And how many of us, having carried out some new and untried treatment, have had this experience of being unable to sleep and of creeping into the ward before anyone else is around, with pulse racing, to see whether the treatment has been a brilliant success or a disastrous failure!

Returning from his first campaign, Paré passed his examinations for admission to the Community of Barber-Surgeons in 1541; soon after, he married and settled down to practice in Paris. However, in those strife-torn days, he was frequently called away into service

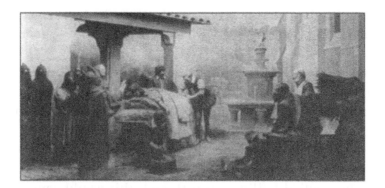

Figure 7.2 **Paré operating on the battlefield at the Siege of Metz.** (Diorama reproduced by kind permission of the Wellcome Institute Library, London.)

and was eventually involved in seventeen campaigns, continuing his shrewd observations wherever he went (Figure 7.2). Ligation of major blood vessels was known to the ancients, and Paré's only claim, as he makes quite clear in his own writings, was that he first applied this technique in performing amputations, thereby ending the torture of the cauterising irons (Figure 7.3). Paré first

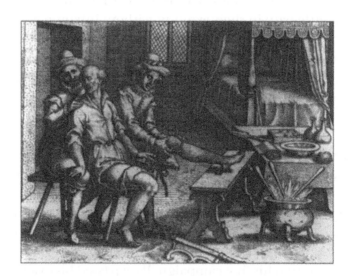

Figure 7.3 **Amputation scene in the late sixteenth century. Note the brazier heating the cauteries. 'De gangreno et sphacelo liber', by Fabry von Hilden.** (Courtesy of the Royal College of Surgeons of England, London.)

employed the ligature in amputation of the leg in 1552, at the siege of Danvillier but did not publish his technique until 1564, in his *Dix Livres de la Chirurgie*, concluding '… wherefore I must earnestly entreate all chirurgeons, that leaving this old, and too cruell way of healing, they would embrace this new, which I thinke was taught mee by the special favour of the sacred Deitie; for I learnt it not of my maisters, nor of any other, neither have I at any time found it used by any'. A description by the master of one such case is worth repeating.

In the year 1583, the tenth day of December, Toussaint Posson, having his leg all ulcered and all the bones caried and rotten, prayed me for the honour of God to cut off his leg by reason of the great pain which he could no longer endure. After his body was prepared I caused his leg to be cut off four fingers below the patella by Daniel Poullet, one of my servants, to teach him and to imbolden him in such works, and there he readily tied the vessels to stay the bleeding without application of hot irons. He was well cured, God be praised, and is returned home to his house with a wooden leg.

So here was Paré (Figure 7.4), at the age of seventy-three, passing down his skill and experience to his apprentices, a tradition we

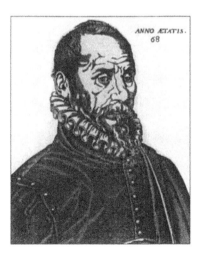

Figure 7.4 **Ambroise Paré at sixty-eight years of age. A wood engraving.** (Reprinted with permission from Keynes G. *The Apologie and Treatise of Ambroise Paré.* New York, Dover Publications, 1951.)

still see today as surgeons teach their residents in our operating theatres.

Paré went from fame to fame and dominated the history of surgery in the sixteenth century. He was surgeon to no fewer than four kings of France, but his practice continued to embrace the humblest soldier as well. Having reached the great age of eighty, he died in Paris in 1590 as he had always lived – a simple, humble man. In his very first campaign he ended his description of the treatment of a gunshot wound of the ankle with his most famous phrase, 'I dressed the wound and God healed him'.

Bibliography

Keynes G. (ed): *The Apologie and Treatise of Ambroise Paré*. London, Dover Publications, 1951.

Hanby WB (ed): *The Case Reports and Autopsy Records of Ambroise Paré*. Springfield, Charles C Thomas, 1960.

8

THE BIRTH OF ANAESTHESIA

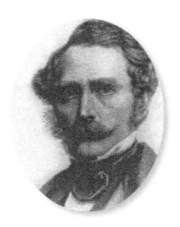

If I were asked to name the most dramatic moment in surgery, it would not be when the clamps were taken off the first heart transplant, nor the first oesophagectomy, or the ablation of any other major organ but a very simple, almost trivial affair – the removal of a benign tumour of the neck. The date was October 16, 1846, the place was the Massachusetts General Hospital in Boston, and the event was the watershed between the past agonies of surgery and the modern era, now only a little over a century and a half old, when patients enjoy the blissful oblivion of anaesthesia.

William Morton (Figure 8.1), the dentist who was to become the father of modern anaesthesia, was twenty-seven years of age. He had been experimenting with ether for dental extractions, and his first patient, Eben Frost, had a tooth pulled out under the influence of ether saturated into a handkerchief on September 30, 1846. The patient testified as follows:

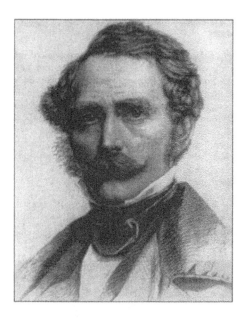

Figure 8.1 **William Morton.** (Reprinted with permission from MacQuitty B: Battle for Oblivion. London, Harrap, 1969.)

This is to certify that I applied to Dr. Morton at 9 o'clock this evening suffering under the most violent toothache; that Dr. Morton took out his pocket handkerchief, saturated with a preparation of his, from which I breathed for about half a minute, and then was lost in sleep. In an instant more I awoke and saw my tooth lying upon the floor. I did not experience the slightest pain whatever. I remained 20 minutes in his office afterward, and felt no unpleasant effects from the operation.

Dr. H.J. Bigelow, son of the great Jacob Bigelow, was attracted by the newspaper reports of Morton's work and went to see him. Impressed by what he saw, he introduced Morton to Professor John Collins Warren (Figure 8.2), then sixty-eight years of age and one of the country's leading surgeons. A few days later Morton received the following letter:

I write at the request of Dr. John Collins Warren to invite you to be present Friday morning, October 16, at 10 o'clock at the

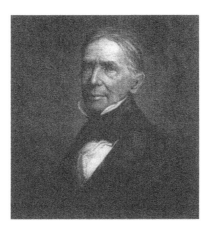

Figure 8.2 **Professor John C. Warren.** (Reprinted with permission from MacQuitty B: Battle for Oblivion. London, Harrap, 1969.)

hospital to administer to a patient who is then to be operated upon, the preparation you have invented to diminish the sensibility to pain.

The letter was signed by Dr. C.F. Heywood, House Surgeon.

It was now only two weeks since ether had been administered to Frost, but already Morton had progressed from a soaked handkerchief to a simple anaesthetic machine. This consisted of a two-necked glass globe, one neck allowing the inflow of air, the other fitted with a wooden mouthpiece through which the patient inhaled air across the surface of the ether in the bottom of the jar.

All the anxieties of a great clinical trial are summed up by Morton's young wife, who wrote:

The night before the operation my husband worked until 1 or 2 o'clock in the morning upon his inhaler. I assisted him, nearly beside myself with anxiety, for the strongest influences had been brought to bear upon me to dissuade him from making this attempt. I had been told that one of two things was sure to happen; either the test would fail and my husband would be ruined by the world's ridicule, or he would kill the patient and be tried for manslaughter. Thus I was drawn in two ways; for while I had unbounded confidence in my husband, it did not seem possible that so young a man could be wiser than the learned and scientific men before whom he proposed to make his demonstration.

The operating theatre at the Massachusetts General Hospital was situated just below the central dome of the old building (Figure 8.3). It is preserved to this day. On the morning of October 16, it was crowded with surgeons and medical students. The audience included both Jacob Bigelow and his son, Henry. The patient was Gilbert Abbott, twenty years of age, who had a benign vascular tumour of the neck. Petrified at the thought of the pain of his operation, he had readily agreed to the experiment. Professor Warren explained to the audience how much he had always wished to free his patients from the pain of operation and for that reason had agreed to the experiment. The time of the operation arrived and passed. By ten minutes past ten Professor Warren picked up his knife and said, 'As Dr. Morton has not arrived, I presume he is otherwise engaged'. (I personally believe that this was simply Morton creating a tradition, which has been handed down from one generation of anaesthetists to another, of keeping the surgeon waiting!)

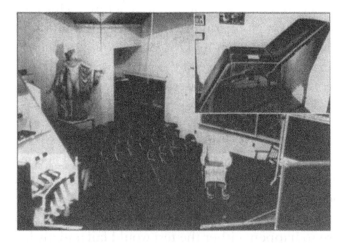

Figure 8.3 'The Ether Dome' – the operating theatre where ether anaesthesia was first used – is still carefully preserved. Inset is the operating table that was employed. (Photograph provided by the General Director, Massachusetts General Hospital, Boston.)

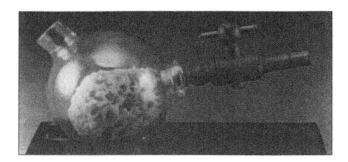

Figure 8.4 **A model of Morton's ether inhaler. The original is in the Massachusetts General Hospital, Boston.**

Just as Abbott was being strapped down on the operating chair, a breathless and flustered Morton arrived; he had been modifying his apparatus up to the very last moment. Warren said, 'Well, sir, your patient is ready'.

'Are you afraid?' Morton asked the patient. 'No, I feel confident that I will do precisely what you tell me'. Morton applied his ether (Figure 8.4), the smell heavily disguised with some aromatic agent to prevent people from recognising it and discovering its secret. Turning to Warren, Morton was now able to say, 'Your patient is ready, doctor'. Many years later Mrs Morton described the scene:

> Then in all parts of the amphitheatre there came a quick catching of breath, followed by a silence almost deathlike, as Dr. Warren stepped forward and prepared to operate.... The patient lay silent, with eyes closed as if in sleep; but everyone present fully expected to hear a shriek of agony ring out as the knife struck down into the sensitive nerves, but the stroke came with no accompanying cry. Then another and another, and still the patient lay silent, sleeping while the blood from the severed artery spurted forth. The surgeon was doing his work, and the patient was free from pain (Figure 8.5).

The operation took thirty minutes, and at the end Abbott agreed that the whole affair had been free from pain. Warren turned to the audience and said, 'Gendemen, this is no humbug'. It took a few moments before the sensational importance of what they had

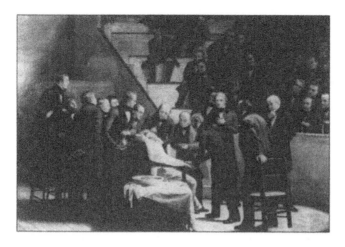

Figure 8.5 **The first operation under general anaesthesia. John Warren operates and William Morton anaesthetises.** (Painting by Robert Hinckley). (Courtesy of the Massachusetts General Hospital, Boston.)

seen struck the audience, who then rushed forward to congratulate Morton, to examine the patient, and to ask him over and over again if the operation had really been painless. Everyone in that room must have realised that they had witnessed an historic occasion.

It was now necessary to proceed to the crucial experiment. The new agent might be effective in the removal of a subcutaneous lump from the neck, but would it work in a capital operation, an amputation? A case was duly scheduled, therefore, for November 7. Before this could be put to the test, a burning ethical issue arose. Should Morton be allowed to administer a secret agent, beneficial though it might be, or should its use be prohibited until its nature was revealed to the medical profession? Warren was prepared to go ahead, his only concern being relief of pain, but the Massachusetts Medical Society resolved unanimously – no formula, no patients. Even though Morton offered to supply the preparation free for use in the Boston hospitals, the doctors remained adamant.

On the very day of the operation the argument continued, with the patient waiting in the anteroom and the theatre packed to the ceiling with expectant doctors and students. Unable to bear the thought of the patient's suffering, Morton quietly announced that his liquid was indeed sulphuric ether.

The patient was a twenty-one-year-old servant girl, Alice Mohan, who had been in the hospital since the previous March with tuberculosis of the knee joint. Dr. George Hayward was to perform the amputation, with Warren and Bigelow in attendance. Morton administered the ether, and after some coughing, the patient fell into a deep sleep. Hayward stuck a pin into her arm and, when there was no reaction, rapidly amputated the leg. As he finished, Alice began to groan and move. Hayward bent over her and said, 'I guess you've been asleep, Alice'. 'I think I have, sir', she replied. 'Well, you know why we brought you here; are you ready?' 'Yes sir, I am ready'. Hayward then reached down, picked up the amputated limb from the sawdust, showed it to her and said, 'It's all done, Alice'. (What Alice said when she saw her leg has not been recorded.)

Scenes of intense excitement were then seen, with the medical audience clapping and shouting with amazement. Morton described the affair modestly: 'I administered the ether with perfect success. This was the first case of amputation'. The patient did well and was discharged from the hospital in time for Christmas (Figure 8.6).

News of 'the most glorious, nay, the most God-like discovery of this or any other age' spread with amazing speed. Bigelow wrote a letter on November 28 to Dr. Francis Boott, an American friend living in Gower Street, London, near the University College Hospital. He enclosed a copy of his son's account of the details of the operations and Morton's apparatus. Boott in turn conveyed the news to Robert Liston, Professor of Surgery at University College Hospital, London, and Liston got his colleague, Dr. William Squire, to obtain ether from an uncle of his, who had a chemist's shop in Oxford Street. The apparatus was assembled, and on December 19, Squire anaesthetised Boott's niece for a dental extraction carried out by James Robinson. The operation was uneventful, and plans were made for major surgery two days later (Figure 8.7).

The patient was Frederick Churchill, a butler who had been admitted a month previously with chronic osteomyelitis of the tibia. At two o'clock the operating theatre at the University College Hospital was packed to capacity. Squire called for a volunteer among the doctors and medical students present, saying that he had only tried the apparatus once before and would like one more

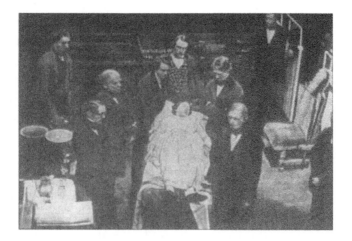

Figure 8.6 **Probably the first photograph of the administration of a general anaesthetic. This is a daguerreotype taken in the winter of 1847 and reproduced from the Transactions of the American Surgical Association, 1897. The original was in the possession of the Warren family. On the patient's left are Dr. John Warren and Dr. Samuel Parkman; on the patient's right, Dr. J. Mason Warren and Dr. S.D. Townsend. The anaesthetist is probably Dr. Charles Heywood, the House Surgeon, who is using a sponge and not an ether inhaler.** (Courtesy of the Massachusetts General Hospital, Boston.)

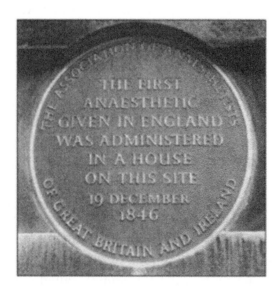

Figure 8.7 **Plaque in Gower Street, London which commemorates the first anaesthetic given in England.** (Photographed by the author.)

rehearsal before submitting a patient to its influence for a capital operation. No one moved. The theatre porter, Shelldrake, was therefore asked to submit to the test. He was not a good choice to try out an anaesthetic as he was fat, plethoric, and with a liver no doubt very used to strong liquor. After a few deep breaths of ether, Shelldrake leaped off the table and ran out of the room, cursing Squire and everybody else at the top of his voice.

Fifteen minutes later, Liston arrived, and Churchill was brought into the theatre by the now sober and recovered Shelldrake. Squire now took the precaution of choosing two hefty students to stand by in case the patient repeated the porter's performance. What happened next has been brilliantly described by Dr. F. W. Cock and is illustrated in Figure 8.8.

A firm step is heard, and Robert Liston enters – that magnificent figure of a man, six foot two inches in height, with a most commanding expression of countenance. He nods quietly to Squire and, turning round to the packed crowd of onlookers, students, colleagues, old students and many of the neighbouring practitioners, says somewhat dryly, "We are going to try a Yankee dodge to-day, gentlemen, for making men insensible." He then

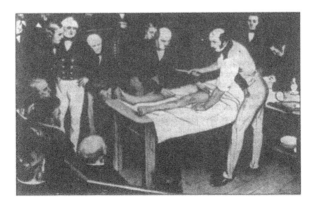

Figure 8.8 **The first amputation under ether at University College Hospital, London, December 21, 1846. Robert Liston is operating in his shirt-sleeves, the ether apparatus is placed on the small table, and the arrow points to young Joseph Lister who was a spectator on this occasion.** (Original painting in University College Hospital, London). (Courtesy of the University College Hospital, London.)

takes from a long narrow case one of the straight amputating
knives of his own invention. It is evidently a favourite instrument,
for on the handle are little notches showing the number of
times he had used it before … The patient is carried in on the
stretcher and laid on the table. The tube is put into his mouth,
William Squire holds it at the patient's nostrils. A couple of
dressers stand by, to hold the patient if necessary, but he never
moves and blows and gurgles away quite quietly. William Squire
looks at Liston and says, "I think he will do, sir." "Take the artery,
Mr. Cadge," cries Liston. Ransome, the House Surgeon, holds
the limb. "Now gentlemen, time me," he says to the students. A
score of watches are pulled out in reply. A huge left hand grasps
the thigh, a thrust of the long, straight knife, two or three rapid
sawing movements, and the upper flap is made; under go his
fingers, and the flap is held back; another thrust, and the point
of the knife comes out in the angle of the upper flap; two or
three more lightning-like movements and the lower flap is cut,
under goes the great thumb and holds it back also; the dresser,
holding the saw by its end, yields it to the surgeon and takes
the knife in return – half a dozen strokes, and Ransome places
the limb in the sawdust. "Twenty-eight seconds," says William
Squire. The femoral artery is taken upon a tenaculum and tied
with two stout ligatures, and five or six more vessels with the
bow forceps and single thread, a strip of wet lint put between
the flaps, and the stump dressed. The patient, trying to raise
himself, says, "When are you going to begin? Take me back, I
can't have it done." He is shown the elevated stump, drops back
and weeps a little; then the porters come in and he is taken
back to bed. Five minutes have elapsed since he left it. As he
goes out, Liston turns again to his audience, so excited that
he almost stammers and hesitates, and exclaims, "This Yankee
dodge, gentlemen, beats mesmerism hollow."

Liston could hardly have realised at that moment that the need
for rapid surgery, which his skill had brought to such a pitch of
perfection, was now to be replaced by the new era, when anaesthesia
would allow calm and unhurried operations.

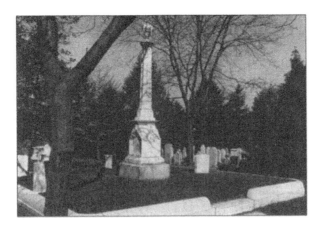

Figure 8.9 **The memorial at Morton's grave, Mount Auburn Cemetery, Boston.**
(Photographed by the author.)

Immediately after Christmas, ether anaesthesia reached my old hospital, Westminster, two or three miles down the road. The operation, however, was far less grand – the scraping off of some venereal warts from a lady of doubtful reputation.

As for Morton, the rest of his short life was not a happy one, although he had the compensation of using ether with great success during the American Civil War. He died in 1868 at only forty-eight years of age. The citizens of Boston erected a splendid commemorative monument (Figure 8.9), the inscription on which was composed by Dr. Jacob Bigelow:

Inventor and revealer of anaesthetic inhalation
By whom pain in surgery was averted and annulled
Before whom in all time surgery was agony
Since whom science has controlled the pain.

Bibliography

Cock FW. The first major operation under ether in England. *Am J Surg* 29(Suppl):98, 1915.

Coltart DJ. Surgery between Hunter and Lister as exemplified by the life and works of Robert Liston (1794–1847). *Proc R Soc Med* 65:556, 1972.

MacQuitty B. *The Battle for Oblivion. Discovery of Anaesthesia.* London, Harrap, 1969.

Warren JC. The influence of anaesthesia on the surgery of the nineteenth century. *Trans Am Surg Assn* 15:1, 1897.

9

THE COMPOUND FRACTURE

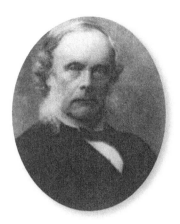

On August 12, 1865, an operation was performed that was to be the watershed between two eras of surgery, the primitive and the modern. Yet, the operation itself was hardly an operation: There was none of the glamour and ritual of the modern operating theatre – no steely eyes gleaming over white masks, no clink of chromium against chromium, no rhythmic purring of elaborate anaesthetic equipment. It was indeed simply the dressing and splintage of a compound fracture. The surgeon was Joseph Lister (Figure 9.1), Professor of Surgery at the Glasgow Royal Infirmary. He was thirty-eight years of age.

Of his patient, Lister wrote, 'On the 12th of August 1865, a boy named James Greenlees, aged eleven years, was admitted to the Glasgow Royal Infirmary (Figures 9.2 and 9.3) with compound fracture of the left leg, caused by the wheel of an empty cart passing

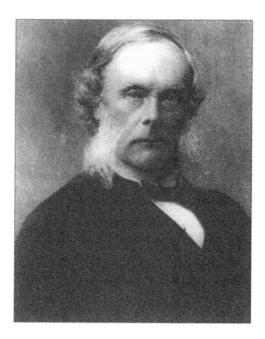

Figure 9.1 **Lord Joseph Lister.** (Courtesy of the Royal College of Surgeons of England, London.)

over the limb a little below its middle. The wound, which was about an inch and a half long and three quarters of an inch broad, was close to, but not exactly over, the line of fracture of the tibia. A probe, however, could be passed beneath the skin over the seat of the fracture and for some inches beyond it'.

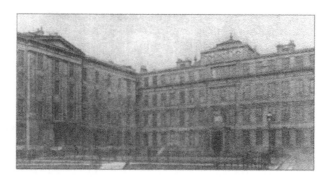

Figure 9.2 **The Royal Infirmary, Glasgow, photographed in Joseph Lister's period.** (Reprinted with permission from Guthrie D. *Lord Lister: His Life and Doctrine*. Edinburgh, ES Livingstone, 1949.)

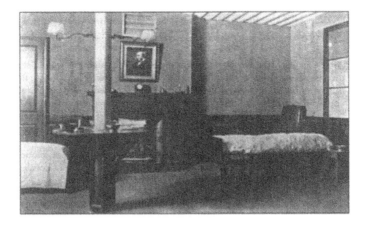

Figure 9.3 **The room in the Royal Infirmary, Glasgow, where the first compound fracture was treated by antiseptic surgical technique.** (Reprinted with permission from Guthrie D. *Lord Lister: His Life and Doctrine*. Edinburgh, ES Livingstone, 1949.)

The treatment consisted of careful application of undiluted carbolic acid to all parts of the wound, which was then dressed with lint soaked in the same fluid. The lint was covered with a sheet of tinfoil to prevent evaporation, and the leg was then carefully splinted. Under the dressing, the blood and carbolic acid formed a protective crust, beneath which, miracle of miracles, the wound began to heal soundly.

After four days, the first dressing was removed. Although the wound was sore, there was none of the usual horrible smell of hospital infection or the other familiar signs of putrefaction, which were expected under the normal course of events within three to four days. Lister dressed the wound again in the same way and left it untouched for another five days. The patient remained comfortable, was eating well, and had little if any fever. At the second dressing, the skin around the wound had been burned by the carbolic acid, so Lister changed the dressing to gauze soaked in a solution of carbolic acid in olive oil. Six weeks after his accident, James Greenlees walked out of the hospital.

The second case was less happy. This was a thirty-two-year-old labourer, whose compound fracture of the thigh produced only a small external wound. He was admitted to the hospital under Lister's care on September 11, and identical treatment was employed. After eleven days, progress seemed to be excellent, and Lister went for a short holiday, leaving the House Surgeon in charge. Unfortunately, gangrene developed, and the leg had to be amputated.

There was now a dearth of compound fractures on Lister's unit, but he spent the time experimenting with carbolic acid in the treatment of leg ulcers and in the use of the antiseptic technique in removing diseased bones from the wrist of a young girl named Janet Forgie. At last a third patient with a compound fracture was admitted on May 19, 1866, a twenty-one-year old man, whose leg had been smashed by a heavy iron box at work. Treatment was successful, as was that of a fourth case, a nasty compound fracture of the forearm in a ten-year-old boy.

Lister delayed publishing his results until a total of eleven patients had been managed by the antiseptic technique. 'On a new method of treating compound fracture, abscesses etc., with observations on the conditions of suppuration' was published in the *Lancet* in five successive issues from March 16 to July 27, 1867. Of the eleven cases of compound fracture, he reported only one death, the sixth in the series, John Campbell, a fifty-seven-year-old quarryman with a compound fracture of the thigh resulting from a large falling rock. There was a six-hour delay and considerable loss of blood before he was admitted to the hospital. After making good progress for several weeks, he died from haemorrhage following the perforation of the femoral artery by a sharp fragment of the fracture.

It must be remembered that, at this time, many compound fractures required amputation, and this procedure was often fatal. The improvement in the statistics on Lister's own service, after the adoption of his antiseptic method, is demonstrated by his published figures. Between 1864 and 1866 there were thirty-five amputations, with sixteen deaths, a forty-six percent mortality. Between 1867 and 1870, when amputations were carried out using the antiseptic technique, forty operations were performed with only six deaths, a fifteen percent mortality. Such results were quite extraordinary in those days.

Before Lister, surgeons hesitated to inflict an incision through the intact skin because of the extreme risk of wound infection, which was often fatal. Even the simplest procedure, like removal of a sebaceous cyst, might be followed by a lethal erysipelas. However, by December 12, 1870 Lister was confident enough to operate on a man whose gross malunion of the ulna had left the limb more or less useless. Under antiseptic precautions and with the addition of a carbolic spray, Lister performed an open osteotomy on the malaligned bone, which, of course, involved transforming the situation into what amounted to a compound fracture. In those days, this could almost be considered malpractice. The wound healed by something rarely seen before Lister – it healed by first intention!*

Enormous new vistas of surgery now lay open. Lister performed an open reduction of a fractured patella, daring to open the intact knee joint and wire the two fragments together; the wound healed. Success followed success as the new antiseptic method became firmly established. While these experiments were going on, Lister was also deeply involved in the problems of arterial ligation. The standard practice for centuries had been to ligate major blood vessels, usually with silk, and then to leave the ends of the ligature long and dangling out of the wound. As the wound suppurated, the ligatures would gradually come away, often helped by a tug from the surgeon and often accompanied by secondary haemorrhage. The brachial artery of Lord Horatio Nelson, for example was dealt with in this standardised manner (*see Chapter 12*).

It is interesting that another surgeon, Sir Asdey Cooper (*see Chapter 2*), tied the femoral artery in a case of popliteal aneurysm using catgut, cut the ends short, and the wound healed by first intention. This was back in 1817.

Lister believed that bacteria-free ligatures might be left safely within the wound, and in 1867, he tied the carotid artery of a horse with a piece of silk soaked in carbolic acid. The ends of the ligature were cut short and the wound closed. First intention

---

* Primary healing.

healing took place, and at autopsy the silk was found unchanged and embedded in fibrous tissue. Following this, Lister ligated the external iliac artery in a fifty-one-year-old woman with an aneurysm of the femoral artery. Again, he used silk soaked in carbolic acid and the operation was successful. He still worried that, even without suppuration, the unabsorbed silk might cause irritation later, and so he turned to catgut prepared from sheep's intestines as a more suitable agent. On Christmas 1886, he carried out his classical experiment on a calf, tying the carotid artery with catgut sterilised in carbolic acid. The operation was a complete success, and when the wound was explored a month later, the original catgut had been entirely replaced. For the rest of his life, Lister remained interested in the best means of sterilising catgut, and some of his original tubes can be seen to this day in the front hall of the Royal College of Surgeons of England in London.

Douglas Guthrie gives a vivid account of Lister at work:

The technique of an operation by Lister ... was very simple. He never wore a white gown and frequently did not even remove his coat, but simply rolled back his sleeves and turned up his coat collar to protect his starched collar from the cloud of carbolic spray in which he operated. Sometimes he would pin an ordinary towel around his neck. The skin of the patient and the hands of the operator and his assistants were treated with carbolic solution (1 in 20). Towels soaked in the solution were placed around the wound. Instruments and sponges were steeped in the same fluid. Neither the operating theatre nor its furnishing were specially adapted for the purpose. The rough wooden floor bore the marks of previous operations, the table was a plain deal board padded with leather, while gas or candles supplied artificial fight when required. One advantage of so simple a method was that the student who saw it practiced in hospital could reproduce it when he commenced practice and had occasion to operate in the homes of his patients. It has been alleged that he was a poor operator, but that is not true. He may have been slow; he had none of the dramatic dash and haste of the surgeon of previous times. But there was now no need for rapid operating. The introduction of anaesthetics allowed the surgeon to proceed with his work calmly, deliberately and carefully. On the occasion when rapid action was demanded, Lister showed that his dexterity was equal to that of other surgeons. As he told his students, 'anaesthetics have abolished the need for operative speed and they allow time for careful procedure,' and he would often add a favourite maxim, 'success depends upon attention to detail.'

I suppose today Lister would have been regarded as an orthopaedic surgeon; indeed, in his whole career, he never opened the abdominal cavity.

Lister was born in 1827 in Upton, Essex. His father, Joseph Jackson Lister, a devout Quaker, was a distinguished microscopist. Lister studied at University College, London, and was said to have been present at Liston's historic amputation of a leg while the patient was anaesthetised by ether (*see Chapter 8*). After qualifying, Lister worked under the famous James Syme in Edinburgh, married his daughter, and was appointed to the Regius Chair of Surgery at Glasgow in 1860; it was here that he laid the foundations of his life's work. In 1869, he was appointed Professor of Clinical Surgery in Edinburgh, and in 1877, he accepted an invitation to the Chair of Surgery at King's College, London. He died in 1912, having been made a baronet in 1883 and a lord in 1897, having served on the Council of the Royal College of Surgeons, and having been one of the first recipients of the Order of Merit.

As far as I know, he is one of only two surgeons in the United Kingdom who has a public monument in his honour (Figure 9.4), the other being John Hunter. It stands, for all to see, in Portland Place in London just south of Portland Crescent, where he lived for many years as Professor of Surgery at King's College and where a plaque commemorates his residence. His monument bears a single word – Lister.

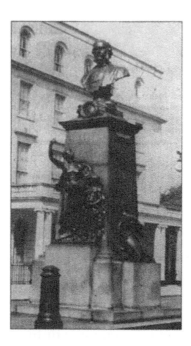

Figure 9.4 **Statue of Lord Joseph Lister in Portland Place, London.** (Reprinted with permission from Guthrie D. *Lord Lister: His Life and Doctrine.* Edinburgh, ES Livinstone, 1949.)

Bibliography

Fisher RB. *Joseph Lister, 1827–1912.* London, Macdonald and Jane's, 1977.
Guthrie D. *Lord Lister, His Life and Doctrine.* Edinburgh, ES Livinstone, 1949.
Lister J. *Collected Papers (2 volumes).* Oxford, Clarendon Press, 1909.

10

ELECTROSURGERY

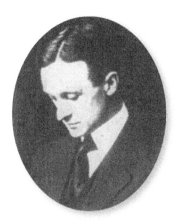

Many surgeons would regard the surgical diathermy unit as the United States' most important contribution to standard surgical technique. Although it was not initiated by Harvey Cushing, there is no doubt that he introduced this apparatus to neurosurgery. The consequent refinements of the apparatus popularised its spread to the other specialties.

Of course the use of intense heat to coagulate and divide the tissues goes back to the very earliest days of surgery. The cautery was certainly used by the ancient Egyptians to staunch severe bleeding from wounds and was much favoured by the Arab school of surgery. The introduction of gunpowder in the Middle Ages was associated with far more serious wounds than had been known in the days of the sword, spear and arrow. The intense suppuration and gangrene that followed bullet wounds were considered to be due to some poisonous substance in the gunpowder, and the surgeons of those days attempted to deal with this by cauterising gunshot wounds with boiling oil. In Chapter 7 we saw how Ambroise Paré conducted perhaps the earliest randomised clinical trial when, as a young army surgeon in his first campaign, he ran out of boiling oil and had to treat men without it, using only a simple lotion. The next morning he found those who had been treated with the lotion had rested fairly comfortably, while those who had undergone the customary treatment were, as can be imagined, in agonising pain. 'Then I resolved within myself never so cruelly to burn poor wounded men'.

Various types of cauterising instruments remained in use over the centuries (Figure 10.1). They were heated at first in the open fire, then, with more sophistication, in a spirit flame, but it was the development of the electric diathermy apparatus that introduced a revolutionary instrument into the surgical armamentarium. The urologists were pioneers in this field. In 1896, Max Nitze developed an operating cystoscope fitted with an electric cautery. The introduction of the high-frequency current enabled Edwin Beer to carry out suprapubic excision and fulguration of bladder tumours, for which special ball, plate and loop electrodes were devised. In 1911, Clark published

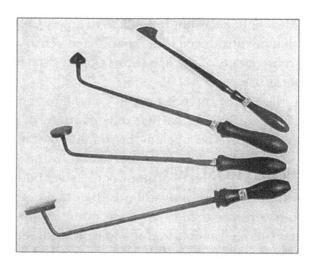

Figure 10.1 **A selection of surgical cauteries.** (Courtesy of the Hunterian Museum, Royal College of Surgeons of England, London.)

his paper on 'Oscillatory desiccation in the treatment of accessible malignant growth and minor surgical conditions: A new electrical effect', in the *Journal of Advanced Therapy*; he had found this method of particular value in dealing with malignant growths such as cancer of the breast.

In the spring or summer of 1926, Cushing, then Surgeon-in-Chief at the Peter Bent Brigham Hospital, Boston, and the Moseley Professor of Surgery at Harvard University Medical School (Figure 10.2), became interested in the use of high-frequency currents to deal with vascular intracranial tumours. The physicist attached to the Harvard Cancer Commission, Dr. W.T. Bovie, had developed two separate high-frequency circuits to aid in the removal of malignant growths, one designed to cut tissues without bleeding and the other to coagulate vessels. Cushing and Bovie collaborated in the development of various loops, balls and steel points, which could be attached to a sterilised handle and used in the application of the electrical current to cerebral tissue.

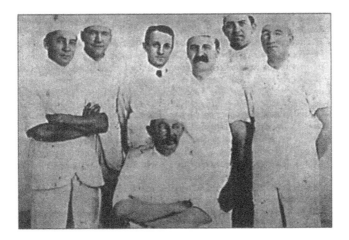

Figure 10.2 Harvey Cushing (third from left) as a young man. This photograph was taken in October 1904, when Cushing was commencing his neurosurgical work at the Johns Hopkins Hospital, Baltimore. Standing: Hugh H. Young, R.H. Follis, Harvey Cushing, J.M.T. Finney, J.C. Bloodgood, and J.F. Mitchell. Seated: William S. Halstead. (Reprinted with permission from Fulton JF. *Harvey Cushing. A Biography.* Oxford, Blackwell Scientific, 1946.)

The first clinical trial took place on October 1, 1926. The patient had a highly vascular myeloma (i.e. meningioma) that had already been explored, but the vascularity of the growth prevented its removal. Cushing's operative note reads as follows:

> This operation was a perfect circus – many ringed. The New England Surgical Association was here and almost every hand was occupied with them. I had persuaded Dr. Bovie to bring his electro-surgical unit over here to let me see what I could do with his cutting loop. This had necessitated re-electrifying the operating room. Dr. Greenough appeared with four or five coughing Frenchmen with colds in their heads, [and] the student who was acting as a possible [blood] donor fainted and fell off the seat. It was a little too much for Davidoff's successor who has been here only two to three days so that I finally had to call in Horrax.... In spite of all this and more, things went surprisingly well. Under novocain a flap was this time turned down with base well in the temporal region so that the scalp could be entirely removed over the situation of the growth. On elevating the flap a large clot was disclosed which was removed by the sucker and a considerable amount of bleeding was started up afresh.... Then with Dr. Bovie's help I proceeded to take off most satisfactorily the remaining portion of tumour with practically none of the bleeding which was occasioned in the preceding operation. The loop acted perfectly and blood stilling was almost complete but whether we would venture to use anything of this kind in the brain tissue itself I am at a loss to know for almost certainly it would cause convulsions.

The next day Cushing wrote to Bovie, 'In spite of the confusion of our many-ringed circus I was delighted to see how well the loop worked. If I could have had it at the first stage, I would have got along as far as I have now in this stage'.

Cushing, much encouraged by the success of his first operation, called back all his patients with what had been thought to have been inoperable meningiomas, particularly those of the olfactory groove and the highly vascular haemangiomas. Although his mortality rate increased to some extent, as a result of attempting to remove tumours that would previously have been regarded as inoperable, his success was striking, and he was able to publish detailed reports on electrosurgery in 1927 and 1928, the latter entitled *Electrosurgery as an Aid to the Removal of Intracrainial Tumours. With a preliminary Note on a New Surgical Current Generator by W.T". Bovie, Ph.D.* To this day the electrodiathermy apparatus in the United States is often called the 'Bovie knife', although this term does not appear to be used (except, I believe, by myself) outside of America.

From his earliest pioneering days in neurosurgery, Cushing (Figure 10.3) realised the vital importance of haemostasis. He had introduced the head tourniquet, which was abandoned when he found that scalp bleeding could be controlled by infiltration with adrenaline combined with traction with a series of artery forceps applied to the skin edges. In 1910, he introduced silver clips, to which his name is still eponymously applied, which could be used to occlude meningeal and cerebral vessels. Suction was introduced to deal with severe haemorrhage, especially deep within the brain substance, and he had his team experiment with a fibrin preparation that might help promote blood clotting.

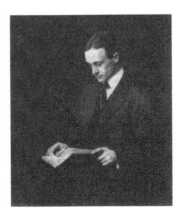

Figure 10.3 **Harvey Cushing (1869–1939). This photograph was taken about 1901.** (Reprinted with permission from Fulton JF. *Harvey Cushing. A Biography.* Oxford, Blackwell Scientific, 1946.)

This first neurosurgical operation using diathermy has a particular fascination for me because the assistant mentioned in the operating note that 'it was a little too much for Davidoff's successor', Sir Hugh Cairns, who was later to become my own Professor of Surgery at Oxford. At that time he was a young Australian veteran of the Gallipoli landings in the First World War, where he had fought against the Turks as a private with the Australians. He later served in France as a junior medical officer. Obviously, the smell of coagulating brain tissue proved too much for him and he fainted; indeed, Cairns used to say that Gallipoli and the battle of the Marne were nothing compared with working as Cushing's resident.

Cushing's publications and Bovie's refined instrument did much to establish the use of the diathermy knife and electrocoagulation in general surgical practice, and today it is found in every reasonably equipped operating theatre throughout the world. In a very wide experience of operating in many different countries, I have only once been forbidden to use the diathermy – at the University Hospital in Timisoara in Romania. I was about to do a demonstration mastectomy, but, when I asked for the diathermy, I was told, 'Do not use it; it explodes'.

Another invaluable contribution to surgical technique – the introduction of rubber gloves – had been made by Cushing's old chief at the Johns Hopkins Hospital in Baltimore, William Halsted. The story is not only interesting but also romantic. Dr. Halsted's operating-room nurse or theatre sister, as we would call her in the United Kingdom, Miss Caroline Hampton, developed an eczema of the delicate skin on her hands from repeated plunging into carbolic acid and bichloride of mercury. The eczema was so severe that she had to transfer from the operating room for some time. Halsted tried painting her hands with collodion, but this failed because the collodion covering would split when the fingers contracted. William H. Welch (of *Clostridium welchii* [*perfringens*] fame, a bacterium responsible for the development of gas gangrene in contaminated wounds) began to employ in his autopsy work a pair of heavy rubber gloves from Germany. When Halsted saw them, he immediately thought of using gloves for Miss Hampton and got the Goodrich Rubber Company to manufacture some.

The original gloves had long sleeves that came up to the elbow, and Miss Hampton found them an immediate success. The eczema disappeared, and Halsted married her.

Joe Bloodgood, who described the 'blue-domed cyst' of the breast, realised the value of these gloves to the rest of the team, saying, 'What is sauce for the goose is sauce for the gander. Why should not the surgeon use the gloves as well as the nurse?' Gradually the use of gloves spread to the entire staff.

Subsequently Johann von Mikulicz, the famous German surgeon visited Halsted, saw the gloves in use, and published a paper on them when he returned home. Mikulicz is often given credit for having introduced rubber gloves into the operating theatre, but this was, in fact, an American innovation – one that was based on the heart rather than the mind.

Bibliography

Cushing HC. Electro-surgery as an aid to the removal of intracranial tumours. With a preliminary note on a new surgical current generator by W.T. Bovie, Ph.D. *Sure Gynecol Obstet* 47:751, 1928.

Fulton JF. *Harvey Cushing. A Biography.* Oxford, Blackwell Scientific, 1946.

11

MINIMAL ACCESS SURGERY

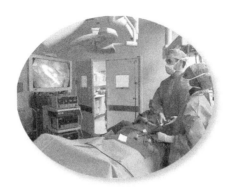

Until comparatively recent years, major operations have usually involved making a large incision through the body wall in order to expose the diseased or damaged organ or tissues and to enable the surgeon to deal with the underlying condition. Many examples of this have been given in the preceding chapters. However, the surgical wound itself presents its own set of problems – problems of pain, wound healing, wound breakdown, wound infection, ugly scars and prolonged hospital stay. Advances in technology in other fields of science have enabled surgeons to devise new, more effective and less aggressive methods of treatment. Indeed, surgeons often lead the field in seizing upon some new and interesting discovery and applying it to the management of their patients.

An excellent example of this is no sooner had it been shown that Thomas Edison's brilliant invention, the electric light bulb, could be miniaturised to the size of your finger nail, the Viennese surgeon, Max Nitze patented the first cystoscope (designed to examine the interior of the urinary bladder), and first successfully performed such an examination in 1879 (Figure 11.1).

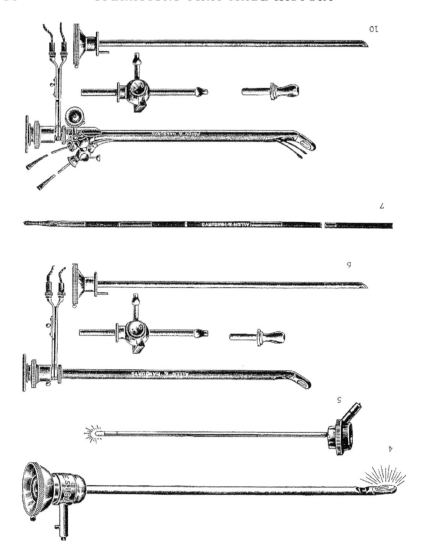

Figure 11.1 **Max Nitze's cystoscope and accessories, patented in Vienna in 1877 and published 2 years later. This marked the birth of 'minimal access surgery'.** (Note, this is Figure 8.24 in 'History of Surgery'.)

Nitze went on to develop instruments to pass into the bladder under vision. These included a snare and a cautery, which he used to avulse or to cauterise papilliferous tumours of the bladder. By 1905, he could report a series of 271 patients he had treated by this endoscopic technique. He stressed that this method was suitable only for benign papilliferous growths and not for infiltrating malignant tumours.

By 1913, Hugh Young, surgeon of Boston in the United States, had devised a cystoscope with a punch attachment, which allowed the surgeon to excise the protruding portion of an enlarged prostate cystoscopically under direct vision. Control of bleeding was a problem until Maximillian Stern of Chicago, in 1926, substituted an electric cautery for the knife, which allowed coagulation of the bleeding vessels. In 1931, Joseph Mccarthy in New York introduced the diathermy cutting loop and popularised the operation of transurethral resection of the prostate, the TURP, especially in the United States.

Following the lead of the urologists, surgeons in other specialties developed metal endoscopes, lit by an electric light bulb, to examine the larynx (laryngoscopy), the trachea and bronchi (bronchoscopy), the rectum and anal canal (sigmoidoscopy – an incorrect term because the instrument rarely traversed the junction between the rectum and sigmoid colon, 'rectoscopy' would be more accurate), the oesophagus (oesophagoscopy), the stomach and the first part of the duodenum (gastroscopy), the pleural cavity (thoracoscopy) and the peritoneal cavity (laparoscopy). Simple procedures such as removal of foreign bodies, biopsy or complete removal of polyps and tumours, dilatation of strictures and so on could be performed under direct vision.

The problem with endoscopes is that, being made of metal, they are rigid and this provides the operator with difficulties in negotiating the instrument through anatomical or pathological tortuosities. For example, a well-known complication of oesophagoscopy or gastoscopy was perforation of the oesophagus, as the instrument pressed against the anterior aspects of the cervical vertebrae, especially in patients with stiff, arthritic necks.

Furthermore, the illumination produced by the tiny electric bulb, although adequate, was far from brilliant.

A revolutionary advance was made by the work of one man, the physicist Harold Hopkins (1918–1994), the father of fibre-optics and fibroscopy.

Hopkins was born in Leicester, read mathematics and physics at Leicester University, graduated BSc with first class honours and embarked on a PhD in nuclear physics. The outbreak of the Second World War, in 1939, interrupted these plans and Hopkins spent the war years designing military optical instruments. After the War, Hopkins moved to the University of Reading, where he was promoted to Professor of Applied Physical Optics. At Reading, his first major work was the invention of the zoom lens. This, he later told me, he first tried out from high up in the stands at a greyhound racetrack! This was followed by the development of the fibroscope – light projected along bundles of fine glass rods, which transmitted a powerful electric light beam with no heat and with high resolution of fine detail. Hopkins patented the lens system in 1959. Sadly, little interest was shown by optical companies in the United Kingdom, but Karl Storz, head of a small German instrument company, bought the patent and began to manufacture endoscopic instruments, both rigid and flexible, lit by this system in 1967. Well before engineers realised the potential value of such instruments for inspecting the insides of their machinery, the medical profession recognised the importance of this new invention, both for diagnosis and therapy. This marked the beginning of modern 'Key hole surgery', which combined brilliant illumination with high definition.

A major advance was the projection of the object, greatly enlarged, onto an optical screen, where it can be viewed, not only by the operator but also by the assistants and the rest of the team, as well as being recorded for teaching purposes (Figures 11.2 and 11.3).

Hopkins was appointed a Fellow of the Royal Society (FRS) as well as receiving many other honours, including Honorary Fellowships of all the British Royal Medical Colleges.

Fibre optic surgical instruments were first taken up by gynaecologists, who were already familiar with the use of the rigid metal instruments for procedures such as tubal surgery. An early pioneer in England was Patrick Steptoe in Oldham. Bt 1968, he could report on a series of 1323 laparoscopic operations, accounting for some 40% of his gynaecological surgery. He published the first book on this subject in 1967 and went on to pioneer in vitro fertilisation with the physiologist, Robert Edwards, resulting in the first successful human "test tube baby", born in 1978.

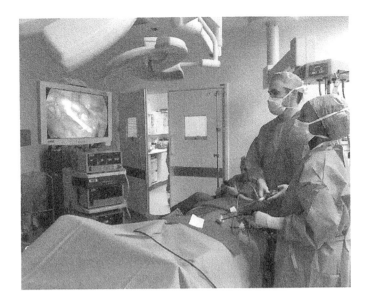

Figure 11.2 **Laparoscopic appendectomy. The surgeon, who holds the operating instruments, and her assistant, who is controlling the laparoscope, stand on the left side of the patient. The monitor and the screen are on the right. Three small incisions are made through the abdominal wall through which the laparoscope and the instruments are passed.**

The first major operation to be performed using this new tool was the common procedure of cholecystectomy, removal of the diseased gall bladder, which previously had been performed by open surgery through a long vertical or oblique incision in the abdominal wall.

The first such operation to be performed laparoscopically was carried out in September 1985 by Erich Muhe in Germany. This was followed by Phillipe Mouret, in Lyons, France in March 1987, the first operation to be performed with video guidance. The first to be carried out in Scotland was performed by Professor Alfred Cuschieri in Dundee in 1988. In England, this first fell to David Rosin at St. Mary's Hospital, London in 1989. David was an old student, house surgeon and lecturer of mine. He telephoned me with the news. I had retired from Surgery just a few months before, so I never had the opportunity of using this wonderful instrument, although I have watched my younger colleagues at work with the

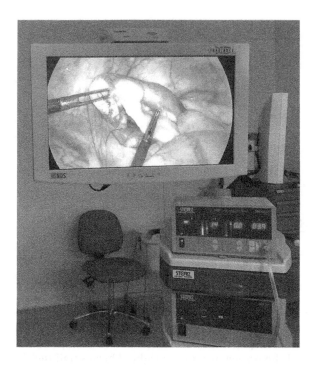

Figure 11.3 **The surgeon's view of the greatly magnified inflamed appendix, seen on the screen.** (Figures 11.2 and 11.3 kindly provided by Ms. Sala Abdulla MRCS at Queen Elizabeth Hospital, London.)

greatest interest and admiration. My good friend Dr. Tehempton Udwadia carried out the first laparoscopic cholecystectomy in Mumbai, India in 1990. The first such operation, as far as I know, performed outside Europe and the United States. The following year he published an excellent and beautifully illustrated textbook on the subject. While in 2001, Jaques Mareseaux carried out a telelaparoscopic cholecystectomy in New York on a patient in an operating theatre in Strasbourg!

Laparoscopic surgery now extended rapidly to other abdominal operations – appendicectomy, repair of hiatus hernias, major cancer resections, and so on. It was found to be of especial value in the new and increasingly common speciality of bariatric surgery – surgery for pathological obesity – which, over the past few decades, has now become epidemic in the Western World. Up to the time I retired from Surgery in 1989, no such case had been referred to

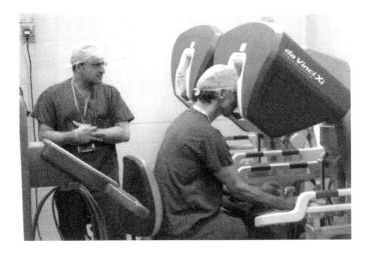

Figure 11.4 **The surgeon sits at the console at a distance and controls the arms of the da Vinci machine.**

my unit or to any other of my colleagues at the old Westminster Hospital. Today, at the same institution, now in its splendid new hospital in Chelsea, there are three consultant surgical specialists dealing almost exclusively with this condition. Open surgery would be especially difficult in having to go through many inches of fat to enter the abdomen, but this presents no particular problem to the surgeon employing endoscopic instruments.

A further step in the story of laparoscopic surgery was the introduction of the Da Vinci surgical system, which, in the year 2000, received initial approval by the Federal Drug Administration (the FDA) in the United States. The name, according to the manufacturer, was chosen because 'Leonardo's study of human anatomy led to the design of the first known robot in history'. The surgeon is seated at the control console (Figure 11.4), which is conventionally situated in the operating theatre, but which can equally be in another room, another building or, indeed, another country. The two robotic arms and hands, capable of a wider range of movement than the human hand (and with complete absence of tremor), are observed and controlled on the TV screen to perform complex abdominal, pelvic or intrathoracic surgery (Figure 11.5). To date, the apparatus has particularly been applied to gynaecological and prostatic cancer surgery.

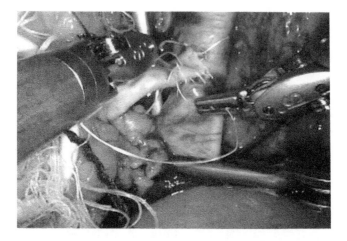

Figure 11.5 **View of the video screen during a renal transplant operation
using the da Vinci machine. The renal artery of the donor kidney
is being sutured to the external iliac artery of the recipient.**
(Figures 11.4 and 11.5 kindly provided by Mr. Pankaj Chandak
MRCS at Guy's Hospital, London.)

Elsewhere, robotic equipment is being used to machine the cavity
in the bone for accurate placement of hip and knee prostheses, for
the accurate placement of a biopsy probe into a cerebral tumour
or for the accurate cutting of the surface of the cornea of the
eye, where the accuracy of the procedure has to be measured in
microns.

An extraordinary development is taking place in the surgery of
major blood vessels with the development of intravascular stenting.
It is now possible to pass a probe along a peripheral artery, the
femoral artery at the groin, for example, and, under X-ray control,
to thread along it a plastic tube and to intubate a major aneurysm,
such as one of the iliac arteries or the aorta itself (Figure 11.6), a
procedure that previously required major reconstructive surgery.
Today, a leaking aneurysm of the aorta, a major and dangerous
emergency, can now be treated in the X-ray department using a
local anaesthetic.

The coronary arteries of the heart can be intubated in the same
way. Thus, a patient with an acute coronary artery occlusion, can
have the obstructed vessel intubated under a local anaesthetic in a
procedure that otherwise would have involved major cardiac surgery

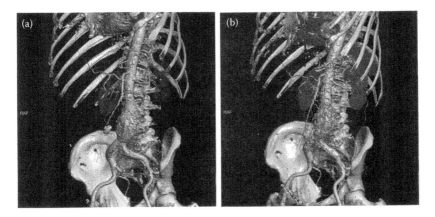

Figure 11.6 (a) Aneurysm of the abdominal aorta. (b) Following insertion of a bifurcated stent into the aorta and right and left common iliac arteries. (Kindly provided by Dr.Tara Mastracci, Complex Aorta Team, Royal Free Hospital, London.)

to perform a coronary by-pass using a heart by-pass apparatus and performed through the opened chest cavity under cardiac arrest!

So, will major 'open' surgery, as we know it today, ever disappear? Since man remains the most aggressive and vicious of all living creatures, there will still remain major trauma. A bullet tearing through the abdominal and/or the thoracic cavity, leaving perforated gut, a shattered liver and/or a torn lung, or a motorcyclist with a compound femoral fracture and major haemorrhage is going to require immediate 'open' surgery, at least until the distant future, as will the patient requiring a major heart operation or extensive reconstructive plastic surgery. But who can tell?

Part III

FAMOUS PATIENTS

12

QUEEN CAROLINE'S UMBILICAL HERNIA

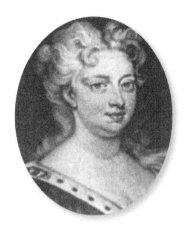

One of the things that we can appreciate from medical history is how immense the improvement has been in the management of everyday emergencies. Let me give one excellent example. Just over two and a half centuries ago, a Queen of England, in her vigorous middle age, died of a strangulated umbilical hernia.

Caroline of Ansbach (Figure 12.1) was born in 1683 and married George (Figure 12.2), Prince of Wales, in her early twenties. She possessed ample Germanic charms: flaxen hair, sky-blue eyes, fair skin and a voluptuous figure. She was also highly intelligent and enjoyed theological speculation. Her husband, like his father George I, was in contrast, rather stupid, although he had a passion for the genealogy of European nobility and an extensive knowledge of the uniforms of all the regiments of Europe.

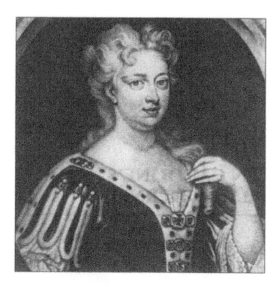

Figure 12.1 **Caroline of Ansbach.**

On the death of George I in 1727, George and Caroline ascended the throne, but by now, seven children and innumerable banquets had converted her to an obese middle age, and her sixth pregnancy in 1723 had left its mark, a large umbilical hernia, (Figure 12.3) which she successfully disguised from her husband for many years.

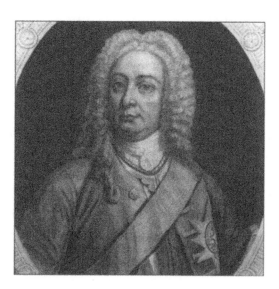

Figure 12.2 **King George II.**

The emergency began on Wednesday, November 9, 1737. Caroline was seized with severe colicky pain and vomiting while at St. James's Palace. Dr. George Tesier, physician to the household, and Dr. Noel Broxolme, of St. George's Hospital were summoned. The usual polypharmacy of the early eighteenth century was immediately put into operation; snake root and brandy, Daffy's Elixir and Sir Walter Raleigh's cordial were prescribed and just as quickly vomited. The Queen was relieved of twelve ounces of blood and was given an enema, which, we read, 'came from her just as it went into her'. Much to the Queen's inconvenience, the King insisted on sharing her bed that night, where neither he could sleep nor she could roll about as readily as she would wish in her pain.

On the next morning, Thursday, another twelve ounces of blood were drawn from the Queen and two more enemas given, which returned 'immediately and pure'. Two additional physicians were called in, Sir Hans Sloane and Dr. Hulse, who ordered blisters and aperients which, again, were vomited.

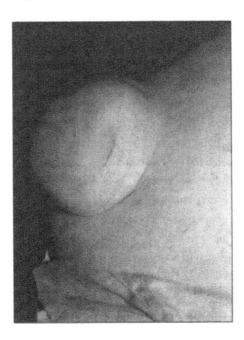

Figure 12.3 NOT the umbilical hernia of Caroline of Ansbach! However, this patient of mine, at Westminster Hospital, had the identical pathology. Fortunately, unlike Caroline, she survived her operation.

On Friday morning the poor woman was bled yet a third time. Early on Saturday morning, the Queen, no doubt by now weak from loss of blood, consented to the indignity of clinical examination; John Ranby, House Surgeon to the King, was allowed to feel the royal abdomen. At once he realised the seriousness of the situation and more surgical consultants were immediately summoned. Ranby advised simple lancing of the hernia and opposed the suggestion of his colleagues that the neck of the navel should be divided wide enough to thrust the gut back into its place, saying that, at this stage, the strangulated bowel would prolapse out of the body into the bed. There is little doubt that, in those preanaesthetic days, and without the advantages of modern relaxant drugs, his advice was probably sound. At six o'clock that evening the surgeons lanced the swelling at the umbilicus and let out some matter but not enough to abate the swelling to any degree or to give them any hope of her recovery.

On Sunday, the lips of the wound were seen to have mortified, and the surgeons, indeed everyone in the royal household, realised that the prognosis was now indeed hopeless. Caroline called George to her side and told him that on her death he should marry again. George was beside himself in misery and with tears streaming down his face, sobbing between every word, said, 'No, I will never marry again, I will simply have mistresses'. This was no doubt a great compliment in the early eighteenth century, when so many husbands expected to outlive one or more of their wives.

Day after day the poor woman's sufferings continued, but she bore them, together with repeated painful dressings of the wound, with considerable courage and without complaint. On Thursday, the strangulated bowel burst, and excrement gushed out of the wound in immense quantities, flooding the bed and flowing all over the floor. When her companions hoped the relief would do her good, the Queen replied, very calmly, that she hoped so too, for that was all the evacuations she would ever have.

Hour by hour the Queen weakened, and indeed the bystanders believed each hour would be her last, but peace did not come until ten o'clock on Sunday night, November 20. Her last word was to her children; it was, 'Pray'.

Today, how often does a patient die of a strangulated umbilical hernia? Even the old and feeble can readily be rescued by the surgical house staff yet, only a couple of hundred years ago, the first lady in the land, obese but otherwise fit, could not be given even the slightest relief by the most distinguished coterie of physicians and surgeons that London could muster.

Ranby, who operated on the Queen, was an interesting man. He was a Londoner, born in 1703, and so was only thirty-four years of age at the time of his royal operation. He continued to serve the royal family for many years and was appointed Serjeant Surgeon in 1740. In 1745, an important event occurred – the dissolution of the United Company of Barbers and Surgeons, whose charter dated back to 1540 and the days of Henry VIII. The barbers defected to form their own company, taking with them the College silver.

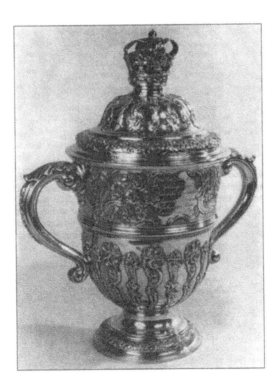

Figure 12.4 **Silver cup presented by John Ranby to the Royal College of Surgeons.** (Courtesy of the Royal College of Surgeons of England, London.)

The surgeons then formed their own company, and Ranby had the honour of serving as first master. This Company of Surgeons later became the Royal College of Surgeons of England. Visitors to the College, to this day, will be shown one of its most precious possessions, a magnificent silver cup (Figure 12.4) on which is inscribed in Latin, 'John Ranby dedicates this memorial, such as it is, to the very worshipful Company of Surgeons on the first day of July 1745, as a token of regard for his brethren'. Surprisingly, there is no known portrait of this distinguished man.

Bibliography

Power D'A. A case of strangulated umbilical hernia. Queen Caroline of Ansbach. *Br J Surg* 20:1, 1932.

13

LORD NELSON'S AMPUTATION

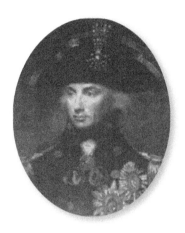

When I was a schoolboy, my hero, whom I shared with most young Englishmen in those far-off days before World War II, was that little 'one-armed one-eyed Admiral', Horatio Nelson (Figure 13.1). I was later to discover, as a surgeon interested in medical history, that the description, 'one-eyed', was not an accurate one. Nelson was indeed blinded in the right eye by sand thrown up by shot in the siege of Calvi in Corsica, July 1794, when he was thirty-five years old; however, the eye was never removed. The cause of blindness has been attributed variously to rupture of the choroid, retinal detachment, or optic atrophy. The loss of Nelson's arm, on the other hand, is undoubtedly the best-known amputation in history, and the story well deserves the telling.

In April 1797, thirty-eight-year-old Nelson, then a Rear Admiral, planned to seize treasure ships that he believed the Viceroy of Mexico had in sanctuary at Santa Cruz on Tenerife, one of the Canary Islands. In July, he set off with four ships of the line, three frigates

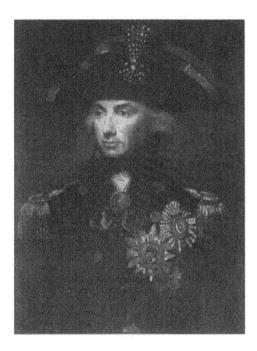

Figure 13.1 **Horatio, Viscount Nelson. Oil painting by L.F. Abbott c.1797.**
(Courtesy of the National Maritime Museum, Greenwich.)

and a cutter, but gales and unfavourable currents deprived the landing of any hope of surprise. Never discouraged, Nelson himself led an armada of rowing boats, setting out from their mother-ships on the night of July 24. The plan was simple: land on the harbour mole and rush the main square of the town.

At half-past one in the morning as the boats approached the mole, the Spaniards opened fire; cannon and muskets crashed out into the night and the losses were heavy. As Nelson scrambled out of his boat onto the mole, his right arm was shattered with grapeshot (Figure 13.2). 'I am shot through the arm, I am a dead man'. He was carried back onto the rowing boat where his stepson, Lieutenant Josiah Nisbet, took the silk handkerchief from around his own neck and fashioned a rough tourniquet around Nelson's arm; in doing so, Nisbet probably saved Nelson's life. Then he seized one of the oars and helped row the boat back from the scene of the carnage.

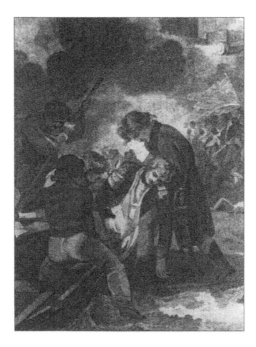

Figure 13.2 **Lord Nelson wounded at Tenerife. He is supported by his stepson, Lieutenant Josiah Nisbet.** (Reprinted from Orme E. *Graphic History of the Life, Exploits and Death of Horatio Nelson.* London, Longmann, Hurst, Rees, and Orme, 1806.)

Nelson was rowed back to his flagship, the *Sea Horse*, but refused to be carried on board for reasons of such extraordinary chivalry that they must seldom have been seen before or since. On board the ship was Betsy Fremande, the pregnant wife of Nelson's Captain. Nelson knew very well that Captain Fremande was still somewhere on the beach and refused to be seen by her in his wounded condition without being able to give her tidings of her husband. He insisted that the boat be rowed on to His Majesty's Ship, *Theseus*, where he refused all help to board. 'Let me alone. I have yet legs left and one arm. Tell the surgeon to make haste and get his instruments. I know I must lose my right arm and the sooner it is off the better'.

The surgeon on board *Theseus* was Thomas Eshelby, then twenty-eight years of age, who had qualified eight years before and had been promoted to surgeon, fourth rate, in 1794. Although young, he had already acquired several years' experience in naval surgery. His assistant, Louis Remonier, was a twenty-four-year-old French Royalist refugee, who had been a surgeon at Toulon Hospital and had permission to serve in the Royal Navy with the rank of surgeon's mate.

The two young men operated in the early hours of the morning in the cold cockpit of the *Theseus*. Eshelby's note in the day's medical journal reads, 'Admiral Nelson. Compound fracture of the right arm by a musket ball passing through a little above the elbow; an artery divided; the arm was immediately amputated'. The tourniquet has been preserved (Figure 13.3). Eshelby's work that night was not finished, he had six more wounded sailors to deal with, including another above-elbow amputation.

It is almost impossible today to picture the scene; the ship tossing on the waves, the assistant holding the lamp, the groans

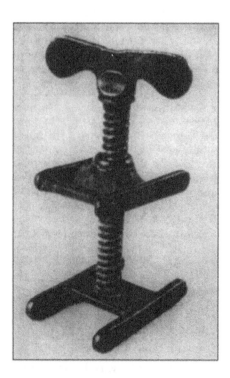

Figure 13.3 **Tourniquet used by Thomas Eshelby in performing the amputation of Lord Nelson's right arm.** (Courtesy of the Wellcome Museum for the History of Medicine, Science Museum, London.)

of the wounded. However, it is not at all surprising to read that Nelson bore the operation with firmness and courage. What upset him most was the shock of the cold knife on the flesh. From then onwards he ordered that hot water should be available to warm the amputation knives when ships went into action and that portable stoves should be supplied to the cockpit in every ship under his command. It is a relief to read that immediately following the operation, the Admiral was given a pill containing opium, perhaps supplemented with a stiff tot of rum.

The next day Eshelby recorded that 'he [Nelson] rested pretty well and quite easy. Tea, soup and sago. Lemonade and tamarind drink'. He had a middling night with no fever. By July 29, the 'stump looked well. No bad symptom whatever occurred. The sore reduced to the size of a shilling. In perfect health. One of the ligatures [had] not come away'.

In an operation performed in the semidarkness by a young surgeon on a famous patient, one is not surprised that Eshelby included the median nerve in the silk ligature around the brachial artery. Nelson suffered a good deal of pain in the stump for many months until he awoke one morning in December of the same year (1797) to find that the ligature had come away in the dressing and that the pain had gone. Following this, the sinus healed rapidly. Nelson, from his lodgings in Bond Street, went to the Church of St. George in Hanover Square, sending a note to the rector saying, 'an officer desires to return thanks to Almighty God for his perfect recovery from a severe wound, and also for many mercies bestowed upon him'.

For the rest of his days, as recorded by his surgeon, Sir William Beatty, Nelson had 'a slight rheumatic affection of the stump of his amputated arm on any sudden variation in the state of the weather. His Lordship usually predicted an alteration in the weather with as much certainty from feeling transient pains in his stump as he could by his marine barometer'.

Eight years later, on October 21, 1805, off Cape Trafalgar, Nelson, pacing the quarterdeck of His Majesty's Ship, *Victory* was shot through the left shoulder by a French sharpshooter at a range of about fifteen yards (Figure 13.4). The ball shattered the second

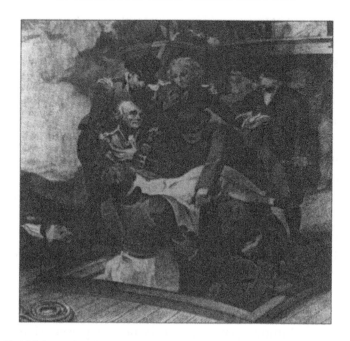

Figure 13.4 **Nelson fatally wounded at Trafalgar.** (Reprint from Orme E. *Graphic History of the Life, Exploits and Death of Horatio Nelson.* London, Longmann, Hurst, Rees and Orme 1806.)

and third ribs, penetrated the left lung, divided a large branch of the pulmonary artery, and smashed the spinal cord between the sixth and seventh thoracic vertebrae (Figure 13.5). To his Captain, his old friend Thomas Hardy, he said, 'They have done for me at last. My backbone is shot through'.

The Admiral was carried down to the cockpit, where he said to his surgeon, William Beatty, 'Ah, Mr. Beatty, you can do nothing for me. I have but a short time to live, my back is shot through'.

Beatty's subsequent report reads:

On his being brought below, he complained of acute pain about the sixth or seventh dorsal vertebra, of privation of sense and motion of the body and inferior extremities; his respiration short and difficult, pulse weak, small, and irregular; he frequently declared his back was shot through; that he felt every instant a gush of blood within his breast; and that he had sensations which indicated to him the approach

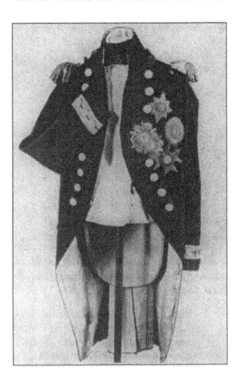

Figure 13.5 **Uniform with the empty right sleeve worn by Lord Nelson at the battle of Trafalgar. The musket ball passed through the left shoulder immediately below the epaulette.** (Courtesy of the National Maritime Museum, Greenwich.)

of death. In the course of an hour his pulse became indistinct, and was gradually lost in the arm; his extremities and forehead became soon afterwards cold. He retained his wonted energy of mind and exercise of his faculties until the latest moment of his existence; and when victory, as signal decisive, was announced to him, he expressed his pious acknowledgement thereof and heart-felt satisfaction at the glorious event in the most emphatic language; he then delivered his last orders with his usual precision, and in a few minutes afterwards expired without a struggle.

In the log of His Majesty's Ship, *Victory* we read: '4.30 P.M. A victory having been reported to the Right Honourable Viscount Nelson K.B., and Commander-in-Chief, he died of his wound'.

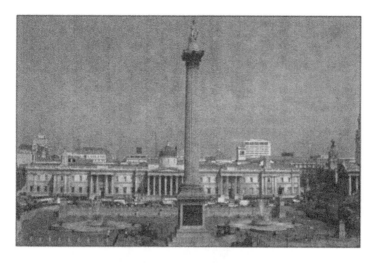

Figure 13.6 **Perhaps the most famous monument in England – Nelson's Column, Trafalgar Square, London.**

Thus perished England's greatest sailor; he was forty-seven years of age (Figure 13.6).

Bibliography

Orme E. *Graphic History of the Life, Exploits, and Death of Horatio Nelson.* London, Longmann, Hurst, Rees, and Orme, 1806.

Pugh PDG. *Nelson and His Surgeons.* Edinburgh, ES Livingstone, 1968.

Warner O. *A Portrait of Lord Nelson.* Harmondsworth, Middlesex, Pelican Books, 1963.

14

THE SEBACEOUS CYST OF GEORGE IV

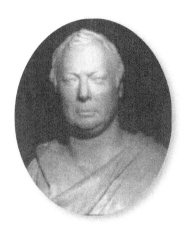

The sebaceous cyst of George IV must surely win the prize for the most minor of any intervention to merit the title of a famous operation; yet, this well-known story is worth repeating for its insight into the surgical customs of the early nineteenth century (1820).

We have already met the surgeon, Sir Astley Cooper of Guy's Hospital, whose dramatic ligation of the abdominal aorta fully merits inclusion (*Chapter 2*). In his account of the present case he writes, 'The King sent to Sir Everard Home, myself and [Benjamin] Brodie to go to Windsor to see a tumour on the summit of his head, which annoyed him from its appearance and was growing larger. When we saw it, it was tender, painful and somewhat inflamed; and we thought it best to delay the operation. The King was much disappointed, but yielded to our advice'.

George IV (Figure 14.1) had ascended the throne only that same year, but he had been King in all but name since 1812, at which time his father, George III, was finally declared hopelessly insane and the Prince of Wales was created Prince Regent. Visitors to London who walk along Regent Street, visit Regent's Park, or admire Regency furniture are paying homage to those interesting days.

Of the three surgeons at that consultation, Cooper has already been described. Home (Figure 14.2), then sixty-four years of age, is probably best known as the brother-in-law of John Hunter. He was surgeon at St. George's Hospital and had been Serjeant Surgeon to the King for twelve years. (Serjeant Surgeon, we should note, is an old title, still in use, for the surgeon who accompanies his King into battle. The last surgeon actually to do so was John Ranby, whose operation on Queen Caroline's umbilical hernia is described in *Chapter 12*.)

Brodie was then a twenty-seven-year-old who had been Home's House Surgeon at St. George's and was now assistant surgeon, having been appointed to staff there in 1822. He eventually became Serjeant Surgeon to Queen Victoria.

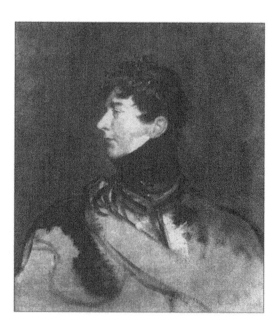

Figure 14.1 **George IV.** (Courtesy of the National Portrait Gallery, London.)

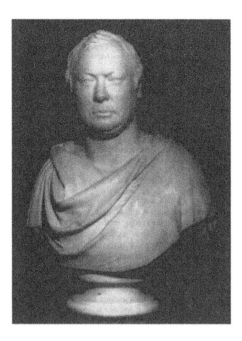

Figure 14.2 **Bust of Sir Everard Home.** (Courtesy of the Royal College of Surgeons of England, London.)

The following year, 1821, Sir Benjamin Bloomfield, who acted as the King's private secretary, summoned Cooper to see the King at the Royal Pavilion, Brighton (Figure 14.3), George IV's favourite residence. He had first visited Brighton in 1783, while still the Prince of Wales, having been told that seawater might be a cure for his glandular swellings of the neck. Two years later, he contracted a secret marriage to the twice-widowed, twenty-five-year-old Catholic, Mrs Anne Marie Fitzherbert, whom he brought to Brighton to stay in a rented farmhouse, a building which was transformed over the next thirty five years into the extraordinary Indian-styled palace that exists today.

At one o'clock in the morning, the King came into Cooper's room and announced, 'I am now ready to have it done. I wish you now to remove this thing from my head'. Cooper was not intimidated by his royal patient and promptly replied, 'Sire, not for the world now, your life is too important to have so serious a thing done in a corner. Lady S. died of erysipelas after such an operation and

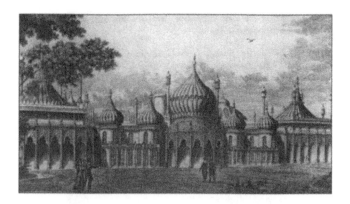

Figure 14.3 **The Royal Pavilion at Brighton, view from East Front. Early nineteenth century print.** (Courtesy of the Royal Pavilion, Art Gallery and Museums Brighton.)

what would the world say if this were to be fatal? No, too much depends upon Your Majesty to suffer me at 1 o'clock in the morning in a retired part of the Pavilion, to perform an operation which, however trifling in general, might by possibility be followed by fatal consequences'. Cooper pointed out that the operation should be done only if other surgeons were present, and mentioned Home, Brodie and his own old chief, Henry Cline. Indeed, Cooper was very anxious for Home to carry out the operation; after all, he was the Serjeant Surgeon, let him have the responsibility of performing this operation.

A few days later all the surgeons and their patient convened in London. Cooper was certain that Home was to do the operation, but the King insisted that it was to be Cooper, who had not even brought his instruments with him and had to borrow a knife from Home.

The King sat down on a chair by the window, and Cooper, assisted by Cline, set to work. He writes:

> I made an incision into the tumour and emptied it of its contents. Then I found it adhered strongly to the scalp .... I with difficulty detached it from the skin without cutting the skin itself. On that side on which Cline stood I begged him to detach it which he did but it took up a great deal of time on

the whole. The edges of the wound were brought together and lint and plaster applied. The King bore the operation well, requested there might be no hurry and when it was finished said, 'What do you call the tumour?' I said, 'A steatoma, Sire' (giving it its now archaic Latin name). 'Then', said he, 'I hope it will stay at home and not annoy me anymore.'

At first all went well, but on the third morning after the operation the King complained that his head was sore all over. Cooper immediately thought that erysipelas had developed and that he would lose not only his royal patient but also his reputation. However, the next day there was a nasty attack of gout in the patient's great toe, and his head had lost all its soreness. From that time on the wound healed favourably. Two weeks afterwards, the King created Cooper a baronet. Having no children to inherit the title, the newly appointed Sir Astley Cooper begged the King to let the title descend to his nephew, Astley, whom he had adopted and educated and who was to follow him on the surgical staff of Guy's Hospital; the King immediately consented to this request.

Today we may wonder that a surgeon should have been knighted simply for removing a royal sebaceous cyst. It is salutary for us to remember that in those days even an operation as trivial as this struck fear into not only the heart of the patient but also that of the surgeon, who was familiar with the fact that even the most minor operation could be followed by overwhelming and fatal sepsis.

Bibliography

Plumb JH. *The First Four Georges*. London, Fontana Books, 12th impression, 1976.

Power D'A. The removal of a sebaceous cyst from King George IV. *Br J Surg* 20:361, 1933.

15

HENRY THOMPSON AND TWO ROYAL BLADDER STONES

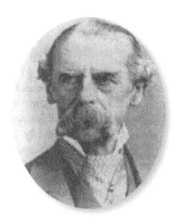

To operate on one Emperor is unusual – to operate on two one might consider an extravagance. Yet, this was the experience of Sir Henry Thompson (Figure 15.1), of University College Hospital, London, who treated not one but two Emperors (admittedly one in exile) for a stone in the bladder. Surely such a duet justifiably warrants inclusion in this volume.

Prince Albert had died of typhoid fever in December 1861, leaving Victoria in blackest mourning and darkest depression. Victoria's father, the Duke of Kent, had died while she was still a child, and she had long regarded her uncle, Leopold I of Belgium (Figure 15.2), as her surrogate father. Early in 1862, Leopold visited his niece at Osborne on the Isle of Wight, but even he could do little to help her. After a few days with the Queen, Leopold interrupted his journey home at Buckingham Palace, but while in London he was seized

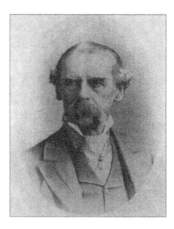

Figure 15.1 **Sir Henry Thompson.** (Courtesy of the Royal College of Surgeons of England, London.)

with all the agonies of bladder stones. Sir James Clark, who had acted as physician to King Leopold in the past, was consulted and advised that the King should be seen by Sir Benjamin Brodie, the Queen's surgeon – the same Benjamin Brodie who, forty-two years before, had been in attendance when Sir Astley Cooper removed George IV's sebaceous cyst (*Chapter 13*). Brodie advised Leopold

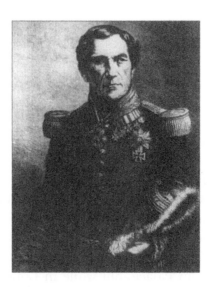

Figure 15.2 **Leopold I of Belgium.** (Reprinted with permission from Ellis H. *History of the Bladder Stone.* Oxford, Blackwell Scientific, 1969.)

to return at once to Brussels and consult Jean Civiale of Paris, whose brilliant work had developed the lithotrite (Figure 15.3), an instrument for crushing the stone within the bladder.

Leopold returned home, and in March 1862, Civiale began a series of attempts to crush the large stone in his bladder. By December, the symptoms were worsening, and Bernhard von Langenbeck of Berlin was summoned for a further opinion. Langenbeck carried out repeated and painful attempts at crushing the stone until his dismissal from the King's service in March 1863.

Clark was again consulted and now advised calling in a young surgeon, Henry Thompson. Clark was fully aware of Thompson's skill, since he himself had been treated by Thompson for prostatic symptoms.

Providing himself with a new set of lithotrites, Thompson arrived at the Palace of Lieken, in Brussels, on May 18. He found his patient to be a fine, distinguished looking man of seventy-three years, standing over six feet in height. By now Leopold was greatly worn by the pain and lack of sleep caused by his stone and not at all happy at the thought of further surgical intervention. Thompson persuaded his royal patient to allow a further sounding of the bladder. The anxieties of a surgeon before an important operation are well mirrored in a letter Thompson wrote to his wife: 'I slept only one and a half hours last night, between 5 and 6:30 a.m. I took too much coffee and couldn't sleep, and then I got thinking about my case and I got horribly anxious about it in the night. No-one knows how anxious, but those who are placed in like circumstances'.

On June 1, Thompson passed a sound into the bladder and detected what he thought to be a stone. On June 6 lithotrity was carried out, and a further crushing was performed four days later.

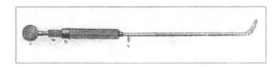

Figure 15.3 **A lithotrite.** (Courtesy of the Royal College of Surgeons of England, London.)

No anaesthetic was used on either occasion, but the King made a remarkably rapid and successful recovery.

The crushed stone was presented by Thompson to the Royal College of Surgeons, London, and there you can see it in the Hunterian Museum to this day (Figure 15.4). Thompson returned from Brussels to London in triumph, with a fee of £3000 in his pocket. A follow-up visit of a week's duration the following year resulted in an additional fee of £1000. His royal patient died on December 10, 1865, but without recurrence of his urinary symptoms.

It was several years later that Thompson realised why his patient had such a smooth postoperative course, compared to the unpleasant sharp fevers he had experienced after the manipulations of his previous surgeons. By now Thompson was aware of the antiseptic theory and realised that his new instruments, freshly unpacked from their greasy, oily, and therefore sterile wrappings, were uncontaminated by previous use on other patients, while those of Civiale and Langenbeck were contaminated by the bacteria of

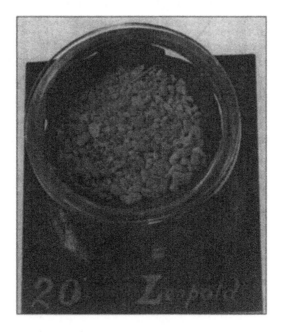

Figure 15.4 **The crushed fragments of Leopold's calculus.** (Courtesy of the Hunterian Museum, the Royal College of Surgeons of England, London.)

dozens of French and German bladders. Thompson received the well-deserved honour of a knighthood in 1867.

Three years later, on July 19, 1870, the Franco-Prussian War broke out. The supreme commander of the French army was the Emperor Napoleon III (Figure 15.5), the nephew of Napoleon Bonaparte. By September 2, the Emperor, with an army of 100,000 men, was surrounded at Sedan by 250,000 German troops. Napoleon III's agony was not, as you might expect, because his army was surrounded by two and a half times its number, but rather because of the stone in his bladder. The first symptoms had appeared fourteen years before, and since then he had had increasing attacks of blood and pus in the urine, with severe pain. By now his condition was pitiful, and he was catheterised twice a day. There were episodes of rigors, his eyelids were puffy, and he would disguise his pale lemon-yellow complexion with rouge. On the battlefield he exposed himself to the enemy's shot and shell without fear, but one wonders whether his bravery was a death wish to escape the tortures of his bladder stone.

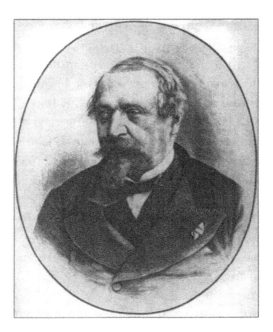

Figure 15.5 **Napoleon III.** (Reprinted with permission from Ellis H. *History of the Bladder Stone*. Oxford, Blackwell Scientific, 1969.)

At the end of the day, he caused the white flag to fly over the battlefield and sent the following message to the Emperor William of Prussia, commander of the German forces in Sedan: 'Sire my brother, being unable to die at the head of my troops, nothing remains but to surrender my sword into the hands of Your Majesty'. Napoleon and the remains of his army were marched off as prisoners of war.

Although the war was to drag on, the fate of France was sealed that day at Sedan. This marked the unification of the German federation under the influence of Bismarck and of Prussia, and the professional historians report that the seeds of the First and Second World Wars were planted on the battlefield of Sedan. As amateur surgical historians, we can only agree with this interpretation; however, we would add that it is likely that those seeds were fertilised with royal urine.

On March 1, 1871, the German troops entered Paris, and it was all over. By March 20, the ex-Emperor was allowed to join his wife, Eugénie, who had already taken up residence at Camden Place in Chislehurst, Kent. Like so many before and since, famous and infamous, they had decided to take up their exile in England. Napoleon III still dreamed of a triumphant return to Paris but realised that with a stone in his bladder he would never be able to appear at the head of his troops mounted on a charger. In July 1872, he consented to be seen by Thompson, who came down to Chislehurst with Sir William Gull of Guy's Hospital, then perhaps the most eminent physician of the day. The two British physicians consulted with Napoleon's doctors, Louis Conneau and Dr. Corvisart, who had accompanied their royal master into exile.

Napoleon refused to have the bladder sounded. In those days, before X-rays, the only way of confirming the presence of a stone was to pass a metal sound into the bladder. The skilled operator could determine not only the presence of the stone, by the clink of stone against metal, but could determine its size and shape with a fair degree of accuracy.

By the end of the year, the symptoms were so severe that surgery could no longer be refused. There was now haematuria after any exercise, severe pain, especially in the perineum, and the urine was thick with pus and deposit.

Immediately after Christmas, on December 26, Thompson sounded the bladder under an anaesthetic administered by Dr. Joseph Thomas Clover (Figure 15.6), 'the most experienced chloroformist of the day'. The presence of a stone was confirmed and a crushing operation advised. Thompson came into residence at Chislehurst for a fee of £2000.

On Thursday, January 2, 1873, lithotrity was performed. Once again the anaesthetic was administered by Dr. Clover in the presence of Gull, the two French surgeons, and Thompson's personal assistant, John Foster. The stone, which was mainly phosphatic, was crushed, and a considerable amount of debris was removed. The next couple of days, however, brought increasing frequency of urination, pain and bleeding, suggesting that a stone was lodged in the posterior urethra. On January 6, under a further anaesthetic, a large fragment of stone was indeed found impacted in the posterior urethra and was pushed back into the bladder where it was crushed.

There was still evidence of obstruction, and a third operation was arranged for January 9. However, on that very morning the patient lapsed into uremic coma and died later that day, surrounded by his

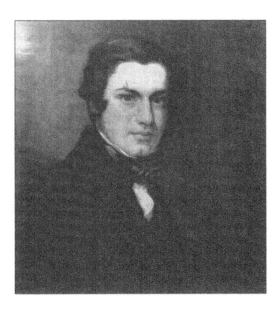

Figure 15.6 **Joseph Thomas Clover.** (Courtesy of the Royal College of Surgeons of England, London.)

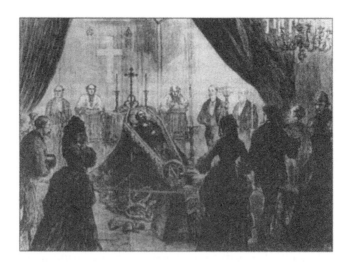

Figure 15.7 **The lying in state of Napoleon III at Camden Place, Chislehurst.** (Reprinted with permission from Ellis H. *History of the Bladder Stone.* Oxford, Blackwell Scientific 1969.)

doctors, his Empress, the Prince Imperial (soon himself to die in the Zulu war) and his priest (Figure 15.7).

The following day, Professor John Burdon-Sanderson of University College, London, came down to Chislehurst and performed an autopsy. The kidneys showed gross pyonephrosis, and within the bladder was half a calculus, weighing about three-quarters of an ounce and measuring one and a quarter inches in diameter. This, too, is preserved to this day in the Hunterian Museum of the Royal College of Surgeons (Figure 15.8).

Two or three days later, Conneau and Corvisart called upon Thompson at his home and presented him with a cheque for £2000; however, Thompson insisted on accepting only half.

Thompson, quite apart from his score of two royal operations, with a fifty percent mortality, was a remarkable man. He was born in 1820 in Framlingham, Suffolk, the son of a lay preacher who was also the local grocer, draper and tallow chandler – an important trade in those days before gas lighting and electricity. Young Thompson was subjected to strict religious discipline and, no doubt as a result, was greatly opposed in later years to compulsory Sunday observance. He left school when he was fifteen years old and started work in

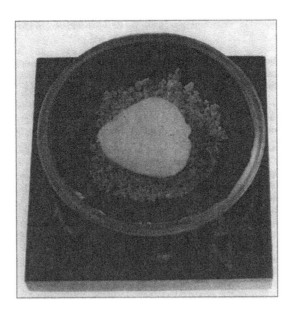

Figure 15.8 **The crushed fragments of the bladder stone of Napoleon III. Note that one half of the stone has remained intact.** (Courtesy of the Hunterian Museum, Royal College of Surgeons of England, London.)

his father's shop; however, young Thompson had his heart set on medicine, and in 1846 he entered University College Hospital as a student, several years older than his fellow students. He qualified three years later and became House Surgeon to James Arnott and Sir John Erichsen; one of his students at that time was Joseph Lister.

Thompson married in 1851, and after a short period in general practice, put up his plate at 16 Wimpole Street, determined on a career in surgery. While his young wife gave piano lessons, Thompson worked to establish himself as a specialist in genitourinary surgery. In 1853, he won the coveted Jacksonian Prize for his essay on urethral stricture, and in 1856, he published 'Enlarged Prostate, Its Pathology and Treatment,' for which he was awarded a second Jacksonian Prize. His work on the prostate brought Sir James Clark, physician to Queen Victoria, to him as a patient, and it was through Clark that he was to meet Leopold I of Belgium.

His enormous experience is confirmed by his collection of a thousand bladder stones, which he had personally removed and which he presented to the Royal College of Surgeons, London.

Unfortunately, this collection was destroyed in the bombing of 1941. Thompson was a man of wide interests. He was a painter who exhibited in the Royal Academy, an authority on porcelain, an early advocate of cremation, a motorcar enthusiast and a successful novelist. He died at eighty-three years of age. Naturally he was cremated.

The nicest story concerning Henry Thompson was related by his former private assistant, Sir George Buckston Browne: 'Sir', he once said to a patient as he lay on the examination couch, 'you have a stone in your bladder'. 'That is impossible', replied the patient, 'I have been reassured by a very rising surgeon that there is nothing of the kind present'. 'Sir, I have risen', was Thompson's prompt reply!

Bibliography

Aronson T. *The Fall of the Third Napoleon*. London, History Book Club, 1970.

Cope Z. *The Versatile Victorian, Being the Life of Sir Henry Thompson Bt. 1820–1904*. London, Harvey and Blythe, 1951.

Ellis H. *A History of the Bladder Stone*. Oxford, Blackwell Scientific, 1969.

16

THE APPENDICEAL ABSCESS OF EDWARD VII

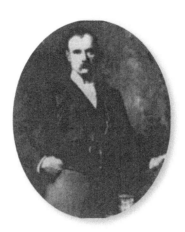

At six-thirty pm on Tuesday, January 22, 1901, at Osborne House on the Isle of Wight, Victoria drew her last breath. She was nearly eighty-two years of age and had ruled for sixty-four years – longer than any other British sovereign. During that time her country had risen to a pinnacle of world power, never before seen in the history of mankind and unlikely ever to be seen anywhere again. No one had waited longer for his inheritance than Edward, Prince of Wales (Figure 16.1), now fifty-nine years of age, whose new titles included that of Emperor of India, King of the United Kingdom of Great Britain, Ireland and the British Dominions Overseas.

A year's mourning was proclaimed, and the coronation was scheduled for June 26 of the following year; however, it was unexpectedly delayed because of an attack of royal appendicitis.

On Saturday June 14, 1902, less than two weeks before the coronation, the King did not feel well but travelled up to Aldershot,

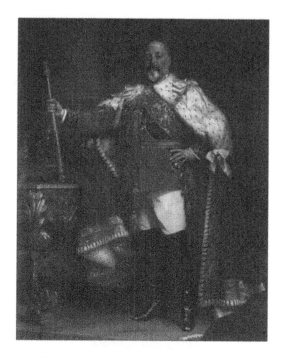

Figure 16.1 **Edward VII. Portrait by Sir Luke Fildes.** (Courtesy of the National Portrait Gallery, London.)

on a typical cold, rainy summer day, to attend a military tattoo. That night his abdominal discomfort and distension became more marked, and by five o'clock in the morning, it was necessary to call in Sir Francis Laking, the King's physician. Sir Thomas Barlow, Physician-Extraordinary to the King, was called in for a consultation. By now there was fever, rigor, and distinct tenderness in the right iliac fossa. Edward, heavily sedated, was transferred to Windsor, leaving Queen Alexandra the task of reviewing the 30,000 troops gathered at Aldershot.

Within the next couple of days, a distinct mass was detected in the lower right abdomen, and, quite naturally, the two physicians wanted the advice of a surgical colleague. Edward stoutly refused: If word got around that a surgeon had been called in for a consultation, people would suspect that some surgical procedure was contemplated, and this might interfere with the coronation arrangements, now at a very advanced stage of preparation. However, Laking, a determined man, sat down at the King's bedside and refused to move until Sir

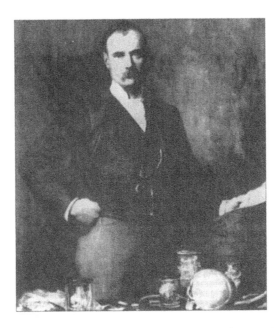

Figure 16.2 **Sir Frederick Treves.** (Courtesy of the Library of the School of St Bartholomew's and the Royal London School of Medicine.)

Frederick Treves (Figure 16.2), the Serjeant Surgeon, was called. After half an hour, the King confessed that the company of his physician had its limits and agreed to see the surgeon.

Treves examined the royal patient on Wednesday, June 18, but by then the appendicular inflammation seemed to be subsiding. Indeed, by Saturday the pyrexia had gone completely, and the mass had practically disappeared. The whole affair seemed to be a triumph for conservative therapy.

On Monday, June 23, the King felt well enough to return to Buckingham Palace. Against all medical advice he insisted on travelling up to London by train and then proceeding by carriage with an escort of cavalry to the palace.

The King wished to be seen by the public, but to the public it was obvious that their monarch was not well. Again against the advice of his doctors, Edward insisted on going to a banquet that night attended by all the crown princes of Europe (all, that is, except the German Crown Prince, kept home by his father, Kaiser Wilhelm, because of his excessive interest in English girls on a previous visit).

Not surprisingly, that night the King's fever returned, as did a large painful mass in the abdomen. Edward was now gravely ill, and Treves, in consultation with Lord Joseph Lister, Sir Thomas Smith and the King's physicians, agreed that immediate surgery was obligatory.

It fell to Lister to explain to the King that his medical advisers all agreed that an operation was urgently necessary. Edward, steeped in the tradition of service to his people, refused: 'I must keep faith with my people and go to the [Westminster] Abbey for the coronation'. This he repeated over and over again as his doctors did their best to persuade him. Treves realised that the time had come to speak quite frankly, and when the King reiterated, 'I must go to the Abbey', Treves finally said, 'Then, Sire, you will go as a corpse'. At this the King rapidly agreed to submit to surgery. Just forty-eight hours before the coronation, the following bulletin was posted outside Buckingham Palace: 'The King is undergoing a surgical operation. The King is suffering from perityphlitis. His condition on Saturday was so satisfactory that it was hoped that with care his Majesty would be able to go through the Coronation ceremony. On Monday evening a recrudescence became manifest, rendering a surgical operation necessary to-day'.

At that very moment a rehearsal was being held at Westminster Abbey. The Bishop of London called for silence, announced the news, and led the congregation on its knees in prayer for the royal patient. Just after midday the King walked into the room in Buckingham Palace prepared for his operation. Frederick Hewitt (later to be knighted) administered the anaesthetic, and Treves explored the right iliac fossa. His patient was obese, and a long incision was necessary. A large abscess was evacuated, washed out and drained with two large tubes. The wound itself was packed with gauze. The whole procedure took about forty minutes.

As news of the royal illness spread throughout London, the royal guests started to slip away to their homes. The vast amount of food that had been prepared for the coronation celebrations could not be preserved in those pre-freezer days and was distributed among the poor of London, who must seldom have feasted better before or since.

Edward's postoperative course was smooth; his temperature was normal within a couple of days, the tube drains were removed on the fifth day, and within two weeks a report in the *British Medical Journal* stated:

> The wound is granulating well, the matter formed is diminishing in quantity and is laudable, but the wound is still deep, and must be dressed from the bottom to ensure sound healing. Sir Frederick Treves and Sir Francis Laking remain in attendance at Buckingham Palace.... The King has been a most excellent patient throughout and has implicitly accepted the advice tended to him.... In view of the fact that sinister stories continue to be manufactured and to be printed, it may again be stated as emphatically as possible, that during the operation no trace of malignant disease was observed, that no suspicion of the kind has arisen since, and that his medical attendants are quite satisfied that His Majesty's constitution is thoroughly sound. His Majesty will leave Buckingham Palace for a change of air shortly, and the date of the coronation will be announced almost immediately.

On August 9, just seven weeks after submitting himself to what in those days was a major and hazardous procedure, Edward went through the full ceremony of his delayed coronation. Indeed, at one point in the service, the King himself raised the frail eighty-year-old Archbishop of Canterbury from his knees.

In the honours list, published shortly afterwards, both Treves and Laking were made baronets, while Lister was one of the first twelve recipients of the new honour of the Order of Merit created by Edward. The King was not to enjoy the throne for many years. By 1906, he began to develop increasing attacks of bronchitis, no doubt aggravated by his very heavy smoking of both cigarettes and cigars. By May 1910, he was becoming increasingly weaker, and on May 6, he collapsed with cor pulmonale. Just before he fell into coma he said, 'No, I shall not give in; I shall go on; I shall work to the last'. The end came peacefully and quietly just before midnight that night.

Treves entered the London Hospital as a student in 1867, just on the eve of modern surgery with its twin boons of antisepsis and anaesthesia, and it was in the London Hospital that he spent his professional life. In 1887, at thirty-four years of age, he performed his first operation on the appendix; it was to straighten out a kink in this organ, hardly a procedure that has passed into the modern surgical armamentarium. By 1901, he had removed a thousand appendices. By forty-five years of age, he was a wealthy man, and retired from the staff of the London Hospital. Following his operation on Edward, he seldom operated again, saying that no surgeon over the age of fifty should continue to operate. From then on, he became an elder statesman of the profession and indulged in his hobbies of travelling and writing.

In 1923, the year of his death at the age of seventy, Treves published *The Elephant Man and Other Reminiscences*, relating fascinating stories of his early days at the London Hospital. In the first chapter, he describes the case of John Merrick, a gross example of neurofibromatosis, who had been under his care in 1886 (Figures 16.3 and 16.4).

I was fortunate enough to acquire a second hand copy of this wonderfully interesting book in 1950, for the princely sum of three shillings and sixpence (about seventeen pence); it became, and still is, one of my most precious possessions. In 1971, I tried to persuade

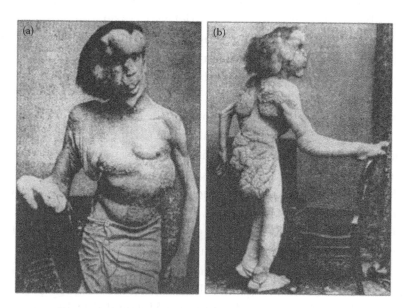

Figure 16.3 **Two photographs of the Elephant Man.** (Reprinted with permission from Br Med J 1:916, 1890.)

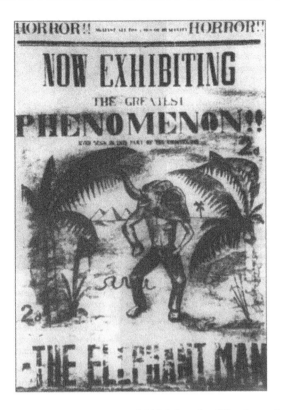

Figure 16.4 **A contemporary poster of 1884 for the 'Elephant Man' in a fun-fair side show. Note that the entrance fee was tuppence.** (Courtesy of the Archivist of the Royal London Hospital.)

the publishers to reissue this book, by then long out of print, pointing out that it was a medical classic, only to be informed that 'interesting as the Treves book is, it is still in some sense a museum piece, and only rarely can one breathe life into a book that speaks so much in the past'. A few yean later, of course, *The Elephant Man* was resurrected as a magnificent play and equally excellent film, and the book itself was reissued in paperback.

Bibliography

Middlemas K. *The Life and Times of Edward VII.* London, Weidenfeld Nicolson, 1972.

Moloney GE. Operation coronation. *Oxford Med School Gaz* 14:141.

17

THE EMPYEMA OF GEORGE V

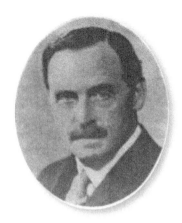

At eight pm on Wednesday, November 21, 1928, a medical bulletin was issued from Buckingham Palace: 'His Majesty the King is suffering from a cold with some fever and is remaining in bed'. The King was George V of England (Figure 17.1), then in his sixty-fourth year. The bulletin was signed by Sir Stanley Hewitt, physician to the King, and by Bertrand Dawson, Lord Dawson of Penn (Figure 17.2), who well earned his nickname 'physician to kings'.

Dawson knew that this was more than just a cold; indeed, he suspected grave mischief. He sent for a young colleague, Lionel Whitby, later Sir Lionel Whitby, one of England's most distinguished pathologists. Whitby has left us an amusing account of his summons:

My services were required at the Palace about nine pm but I could not be located. I was, in fact, out to dinner, and for once (never again!) had failed to leave my whereabouts. When I returned home about midnight, after a good dinner, Lord

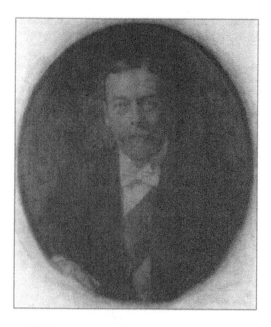

Figure 17.1 **George V. Portrait by Lance Calkin.** (Courtesy of the National Portrait Gallery, London.)

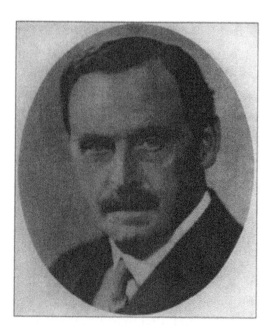

Figure 17.2 **Lord Dawson of Penn.** (Reprinted from Watson F. *Dawson of Penn, a Biography.* London. Chatto and Windus, 1950.)

Dawson's chauffeur was patiently waiting at my door. He had been there for two hours. Needless to say I was at the Palace in record time, to be received by a quite unperturbed Lord Dawson who said, 'I am so glad you have come. I have had a job to avoid sending for somebody else but I said you were the only man I wanted'.

Whitby gives an interesting account of how he had passed his preliminary tests with Dawson. He had first come to the notice of the great man three years before when he had been qualified for only two years but had identified the first case of abortus fever in England. Whitby records that he was summoned to Dawson's consulting rooms:

> ... with everything in readiness for a complete bacteriological, haematological and chemical overhaul. To my surprise my patient was none other than Lord Dawson himself, and after taking his history I proceeded to take my samples, which provided me with about two days, work. Needless to say, everything was normal. It is my opinion that Lord Dawson knew this at the time, and that the purpose of my visit was not his own investigation but rather that he might see the technique, endure the unpleasant procedures and so judge for himself my manner of handling a patient, needling veins and other painful manoeuvres. I must add that he insisted upon paying me full fees for the work which I had done – to my great embarrassment.

How many of us today, I wonder, are so fussy about choosing a pathologist? On November 23, Whitby's blood cultures grew profuse streptococci. Graham Hodgson of King's College Hospital, at that time another one of Dawson's bright young men, brought a rather cumbersome X-ray machine to the palace on a lorry, the first time X-rays had been taken outside a hospital. His films of the chest confirmed the clinical diagnosis of a right lower lobe pneumonia.

Few practising doctors today are old enough to remember those presulphonamide, preantibiotic times when pneumonia signified a desperate struggle against death, and careful nursing – and prayer – were almost the only weapons available to the medical profession.

The King's condition progressively deteriorated. The bulletin on December 1 reported 'a decline in the strength of the heart', and Edward, Prince of Wales, was recalled from East Africa, where he was shooting big game. If anything happened, he would immediately succeed to the throne.

Two days later, two more distinguished physicians were called in to give their weighty help, Sir Farquhar Buzzard and Sir Humphrey Rolleston, Regius Professors of Medicine at the Universities of Oxford and Cambridge, respectively. They could do little except to agree to the palliatives for the royal patient's pleuritic pain, oxygen for his dyspnoea, and skilled nursing to encourage the very little nourishment the King could take from the proffered feeding cups. Much of the time he lay in a muttering delirium interspersed with short periods of disturbed sleep. This was, of course, long before the days of nasogastric or intravenous feeding in patients in such a condition.

By December 11, the Prince of Wales had arrived home to be with Queen Mary and the rest of the Royal Family and the next day, now the twenty-second day of illness, it seemed as if it might well be the end. That afternoon Dawson entered the sickroom, looked at the unconscious King and decided to make yet a further attempt to discover pus in the chest. Asking Sister Catherine Black, the nurse on duty, for a syringe, he promptly drew off sixteen ounces of pus from the right pleural cavity.

Dawson immediately summoned Sir Hugh Rigby (Figure 17.3), the Serjeant Surgeon to the King, and Dr. Francis Shipway, the anaesthetist. A rib resection was performed at ten minutes before eight o'clock that evening, and the empyema drained.

Rigby had spent his professional life at the London Hospital, apart from service in the South African War and as consultant surgeon, with the rank of colonel, to the British Expeditionary Force in France in the First World War. He wrote little and did not take part in many professional activities but had a reputation as a sound surgeon and a modest and upright man.

Meantime, hundreds of people from all over the world were sending remedies and suggestions for treatment to the palace.

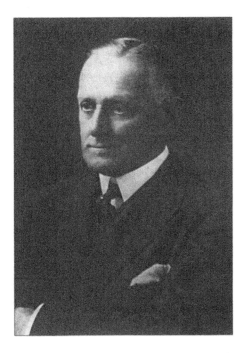

Figure 17.3 **Sir Hugh Mallinson Rigby, Bart.t K.C.V.O. Surgeon to the London Hospital, 1902–1944; demonstrator of anatomy, 1901–1903; teacher of elementary clinical surgery, 1903–1908; and demonstrator of surgical pathology, 1909–1912.** (Courtesy of the Royal London Medical College.)

They included a secret ointment offered by a gypsy family, a hand-knitted chest protector from Scotland containing dried herbs 'guaranteed to draw out the worst inflammations', and all sorts of household cough medicines.

By the beginning of February, the King was fit enough to be sent to Bognor – on the south coast – for convalescence. Bognor was then a small seaside town, but after its royal visitor, it earned the title 'Bognor Regis' and blossomed into considerable popularity. For the first time since the beginning of the illness, Dawson was free from having to visit his King every day. Honours were distributed to the members of the team – both doctors and nurses. Rigby was created a baronet, Shipway was knighted and Dawson was made a privy counsellor.

However, empyema in those days, much more even than now, was a difficult thing to heal. In May, Dawson at last took a well-earned holiday in Tangier, only to receive an urgent telegram through the British consul recalling him to Windsor, which he reached in a day and a half by sea, rail, air, and road. A local abscess had formed at the site of the operation, but fortunately this burst spontaneously.

On July 7, a national thanksgiving service was held at Westminster Abbey. Little did the cheering crowds realise that their King had a discharging open wound on his posterior chest wall.

After further chest X-rays, it was obvious that definitive drainage of the residual abscess must be carried out. There is no truth at all in the rumour, which persists to this day, that Professor Ferdinand Sauerbruch was secretly summoned to London to put things right. In fact, on July 10, Wilfred Trotter (Figure 17.4) of University College Hospital was called into a grand consultation, and on July 15, with Shipway once again as the anaesthetist, Trotter and Rigby drained the chronic cavity. All went well, and next morning the King had tea, toast and an egg for breakfast.

Wilfred Trotter, who at that time was surgeon to the King and who succeeded Rigby as Serjeant Surgeon in 1932, was a

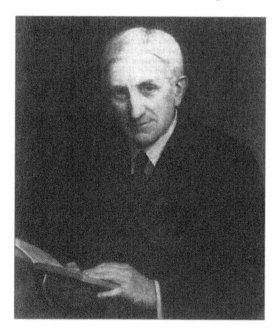

Figure 17.4 **Wilfred Trotter.** (Courtesy of the Royal College of Surgeons of England, London.)

remarkable man. Frail looking, quiet, soft-spoken, and stooping as a result of a childhood disease of the spine, he was nevertheless a magnificent surgeon who made great contributions to the intricate problem of cancer of the larynx and pharynx. One observer wrote, 'It was perfect joy to watch him remove a simple appendix, the knife handled as [Johannes] Vermeer must have wielded his brush, the needle with the skill of an embroidress, and above all, the surpassing gentleness of his manipulation'. He eschewed all honours but was very proud of his election as a Fellow of the Royal Society, in recognition of his scientific work.

The King survived this serious illness for another seven years and was able to undertake with Queen Mary the arduous duties of the Silver Jubilee celebrations in 1935. The end came in January 1936, from the same disease that killed his father, Edward VII – cor pulmonale resulting from his chronic bronchitis (he too was a heavy smoker). Dawson was once again in charge of the case. The last bulletin, issued on the evening radio news broadcast by the British Broadcasting Corporation, was composed by Dawson on the back of a menu card at Sandringham Palace. The words were to become famous: 'The King's life is moving peacefully towards its close'. I was ten years of age at the time, but I can remember clearly the solemn impact of those words.

Dawson died in 1945. His long life crossed two centuries and spanned two world wars. When he was a medical student, the first electric lights were beginning to appear on the streets of London. He died a few weeks before the first atom bomb was dropped. He trained at, and passed his professional days in, the London Hospital Medical College in the poorest section of the East End, where one young cockney patient said to another in Dawson's ward, 'You'll be all right, your doctor looks after me – and the King'.

Bibliography

Power D'A, Le Fanu WR. *Lives of the Fellows of the Royal College of Surgeons of England, 1930 to 1951*. London, The Royal College of Surgeons of England, 1953.

Watson F. *Dawson of Penn, a Biography*. London. Chatto and Windus, 1950.

18

THE PNEUMONECTOMY OF
GEORGE VI

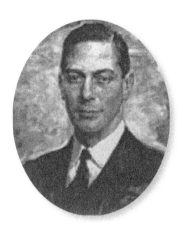

For my last story, I turn to my old hospital and write of senior colleagues, some now dead, others retired, who were involved in a royal operation. The patient was George VI (Figure 18.1), a sovereign still held dear in the heart of every British citizen born more than sixty years ago.

Prince Albert George was born in 1895, a year after his eldest brother. There were four more children: Mary, the Princess Royal; Henry, Duke of Gloucester; George, Duke of York; and John, the youngest, who was to die in his early teens. From the beginning, it was David, soon to be made Prince of Wales, who was to succeed to the throne.

Prince Albert, like his father before him, had a career in the navy. His constitution was never robust, and as a naval cadet at Osborne he had a severe attack of pneumonia. From his early years, also, he was plagued with a severe stammer which, with the help of an

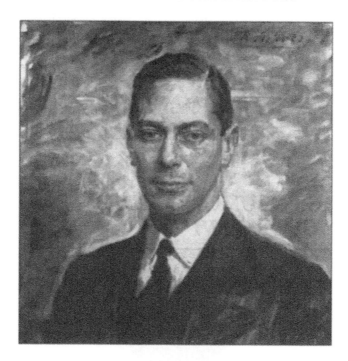

Figure 18.1 **King George VI. Portrait by Reginald Grenville Eves.** (Courtesy of the National Portrait Gallery, London.)

Australian speech therapist, he did much to correct. In the First World War, he served as a naval officer, was second in command in the fore-turret of His Majesty's Ship, Collingwood, at the battle of Jutland but had to be operated on in 1917 for a duodenal ulcer; presumably in those days he would have had a gastrojejunostomy. In 1920, Albert became His Royal Highness the Duke of York, and three years later he married Lady Elizabeth Bowes-Lyon, who came from a distinguished old Scottish family. Their first daughter, Elizabeth – now, of course, Queen Elizabeth II – was born in 1926, and Princess Margaret Rose was born in 1930.

The calm was shattered in December 1936, when brother David, who had come to the throne as Edward VIII only months before, announced his abdication as the only solution to a constitutional crisis brought about by his wish to marry a woman who was not only a commoner but also twice divorced. Albert, as next in succession, found himself, unprepared and to his surprise, ascending the throne as George VI.

Within three years the Second World War was declared, and it was in the following years that the King endeared himself to the people of his country and his Commonwealth. Together with Elizabeth, he stayed in London during the height of the blitzkrieg, although Buckingham Palace was badly damaged on several occasions. The royal couple constantly visited troops, factories, hospitals and bomb victims. After her own home had been damaged, the Queen confessed, 'I'm almost comforted that we've been hit. It makes me feel I can look the blitzed East End in the face. They are so brave'.

Soon after the war George developed signs of severe arterial impairment of the legs. Like his father, George V and grandfather Edward VII, he was a heavy cigarette smoker. By March 1949, surgery was necessary, and a right lumbar sympathectomy was performed by Professor James Learmonth of the University of Edinburgh and Professor James Paterson Ross of St. Bartholomew's Hospital. The King made a good recovery, and both of his surgeons were knighted.

The King undertook a number of public engagements in 1950, and early in 1951, but those who saw him realised he was still a very sick man. On June 1, 1951, a bulletin was issued by the King's physicians: 'The King has been confined to his room for the past week with an attack of influenza. There is now a small area of catarrhal inflammation in the lung, but the constitutional disturbance is slight'. The bulletin was signed by the King's physicians, Sir Daniel Davies, Sir Horace Evans, Dr. G. (later Sir Geoffrey) Marshall, and Sir John Weir. On June 4, the next bulletin announced, 'The catarrhal inflammation in the King's lung has not entirely disappeared, though His Majesty's general condition has improved. A period of complete rest will be essential to His Majesty's recovery, and on the advice of his doctors he has reluctantly decided to cancel all his public engagements for at least four weeks'.

A period of convalescence at Balmoral Castle in Scotland produced no real improvement. Further X-rays of the chest were taken, and it was obvious that the King had to return at once to London. A bulletin dated September 18 read, 'During the King's recent illness a series of examinations have been carried out, including radiology and bronchoscopy. These investigations now

show structural changes to have developed in the lung. His Majesty
has been advised to stay in London for further treatment'. There
were now new names on the bulletin, including those of Dr. Peter
Kerley, radiologist to Westminster Hospital and Clement Price-
Thomas (Figure 18.2), senior surgeon at Westminster and surgeon

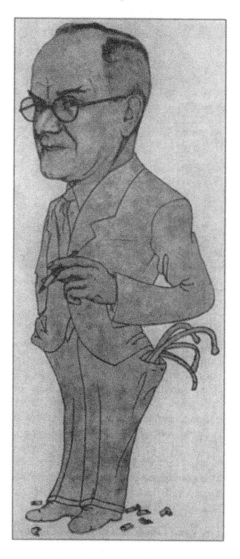

Figure 18.2 **Caricature of Sir Clement ('Clem') Price-Thomas, K.C.V.O.
Notice the characteristic collection of cigarette stubs at his feet.**
(Reprinted with permission from Broadway, the magazine of the
Westminster medical students.)

to the Brompton Hospital for Diseases of the Lung. The bulletin three days later stated, 'The condition of the King's lung gives cause for concern. In view of the structural changes referred to in the last bulletin we have advised His Majesty to undergo an operation in the near future. This advice the King has accepted'.

The word cancer was never used in any bulletin before or after the operation, but there could be few doctors, indeed, few members of the lay public, who doubted the serious nature of the 'structural changes'.

Meanwhile, there was frantic activity at Westminster Hospital and at Buckingham Palace; the operating theatre staff (Figure 18.3) were converting a room at the palace into the exact replica of Price-Thomas's operating theatre at Westminster. Leading them was Sister Sarah Minter, the theatre superintendent, together with Sister Vera Ream (who later married an ear, nose and throat surgeon), staff nurse Audrey Patterson (later a senior nursing officer at Westminster), and staff nurse Hilda Ross (who later married an American lawyer).

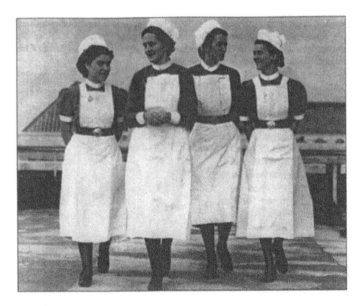

Figure 18.3 **Clement Price-Thomas's theatre nursing staff. From left to right, Hilda Ross (staff nurse), Vera Ream (theatre sister), Sarah Minter (theatre superintendent), and Audrey Patterson (staff nurse).**

The surgeon's two senior residents, Charles Drew and Peter Jones, not only assisted at the operation but also lived in the palace to look after their royal patient (Figure 18.4). His anaesthetists, Robert Mackray and Cyril Scurr, ensured that every piece of anaesthetic equipment was in good working order. Joseph Humble, the haematologist, made blood available. Everything was done to

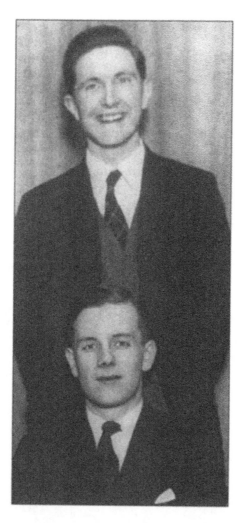

Figure 18.4 **The two surgical registrars who assisted Price-Thomas at the palace. Charles Drew (standing) and Peter Jones (sitting). Both were subsequently appointed consultant thoracic surgeons to Westminster Hospital.** (Photograph kindly provided by Dr. Peter Hansell.)

ensure that the operation would be like any routine thoracotomy at Westminster Hospital.

On the morning of Sunday, September 23, a pneumonectomy was performed – a routine operation carried out by the routine team of Westminster Hospital. The only untoward event during the day was that of Price-Thomas, who upon driving out of the palace forecourt, with his mind very far away, collided with another vehicle; the police refused to prosecute. A bulletin issued that evening reported, 'The King underwent an operation for lung resection this morning. Whilst anxiety must remain for some days, His Majesty's immediate postoperative condition is satisfactory'.

In the New Year's honours list, published in the London Gazette on January 1, 1952, were the names of the radiologist, anaesthetists and surgical residents of Westminster, but Price-Thomas had already been appointed a Knight Commander of the Royal Victorian Order.

A visitor to Westminster Hospital chapel can see the commemorative stained glass window (Figure 18.5) to King George VI, who became our patron; Queen Elizabeth, the Queen Mother, remains our patron today. For many years the operating table (Figure 18.6) used at Buckingham Palace was in daily employment in operating theatres at the Westminster, suitably decorated by a plaque attached to its plinth. It was only when it was far beyond repair that it was trundled into the hospital museum for safekeeping.

Price-Thomas (Clem to all his friends) was born in Wales in 1893 and never lost either his Welsh accent or his Welsh patriotism. After serving as a private in the Army Medical Corps during the First World War, seeing action at Gallipoli against the Turks, he qualified at Westminster Hospital in 1921. He learned his thoracic surgery from that early pioneer, Tudor Edwards, another Welshman, and at thirty-four years of age was appointed to the staff of this hospital. He also served as consultant to the Brompton Hospital for Diseases of the Chest and was consultant chest surgeon to the army and the air force. He was one of that small group of pioneers who established the science and art of thoracic surgery. He was a heavy smoker and always carried a packet of fifty cigarettes in his pocket. It was almost inevitable that he should develop the

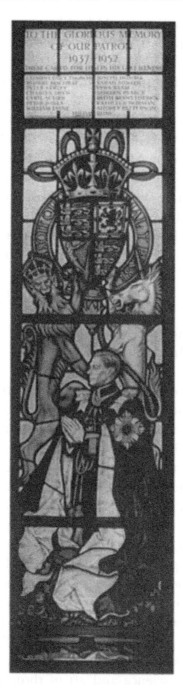

Figure 18.5 The commemorative stained glass window to King George VI in the chapel of Westminster Hospital.

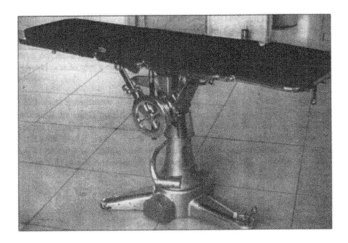

Figure 18.6 **The 'Royal' operating table, which was used by myself and other members of the surgical staff for many years in the main theatres of Westminster Hospital. The plaque on its base commemorates its use in Buckingham Palace.**

disease, for the treatment of which he had become famous. Sure enough, he underwent successful resection of a carcinoma of the lung performed by those same two men whom he had trained and who had assisted him at the palace, Charles Drew and Peter Jones. Thanks to an early diagnosis and their skill he survived for many years and died peacefully in 1973 at seventy-nine years of age.

Following his pneumonectomy, the King made a steady and uneventful recovery. By Christmas he was able to make his usual sovereign's message, broadcast on the radio – not 'live' this time, but transmitted as a tape recording. People listening to the broadcast throughout the British Commonwealth were moved by his words of simple faith delivered in a now slow and husky voice.

At the end of January, Princess Elizabeth and Prince Philip set out in place of the King on a tour of Africa that was to lead to Australia and New Zealand. At the London airport, the King stood on the cold and windy tarmac watching the aircraft long after take-off until it disappeared into the sky.

He returned to Sandringham in Norfolk, probably his favourite home, and was able to enjoy walking in the countryside. On February 5, after a peaceful day, he retired to bed at his usual hour and was found dead the next morning when his valet went into the bedroom with a cup of tea. He was fifty-six years of age.

Princess Elizabeth, at the age of twenty-five, was summoned back from Kenya to begin Britain's second Elizabethan era. The Duke of Windsor, who had handed over the heavy burden of the throne to his younger brother, arrived to take his place beside the three other Royal Dukes – Edinburgh, Gloucester and Kent. Dressed in the uniform of Admiral of the Fleet, he followed the coffin of his brother through the streets of London and Windsor.

Bibliography

Bulletins on the King's health. *Br Med J* 2:793, 1951.
Obituary 'King George VI'. *Br Med J* 1:386, 1952.
Talbot G. *Queen Elizabeth the Queen Mother.* London, Country Life Books, 1978.

19

ENVOI

And so the pleasant task of recording some of my favourite stories has come to an end. From the boiling oil in the days of Ambroise Paré to the 6-mercaptopurine of the transplant surgeons; from the bravery of Caroline of Ansbach to the courage of George VI (Figure 19.1).

What of the future? The first operation in outer space must surely take place one day and will no doubt be relayed world-wide on whatever viewing apparatus people will be wearing on their wrists at the time. The first 'Famous Operation' to be performed by a female surgeon is still, as far as I know, a thing of the future. This in spite of the fact that more and more women are now surgeons; many occupy senior positions and there has already been the first female President of the Royal College of Surgeons of England (Dame Claire Marx, DBE).

However, is there any value in reading about surgical operations of the past? Should we not agree with Henry Ford that 'History is bunk'? To my mind, no. I believe that there is much to be learned from our surgical forefathers and the traditions that they engendered. I personally derive considerable comfort and inspiration from the past. When I used to complain about the working conditions in my operating theatre, a few moments remembering Thomas F.shelby amputating Nelson's arm by candlelight in the swaying cockpit of His Majesty's Ship *Theseus* soon restored my sense of values. When there were problems getting equipment, I thought of Robert Liston, at University College Hospital, who, within days of hearing about ether, had the drug obtained, the apparatus built and the first patient under its influence on the operating table.

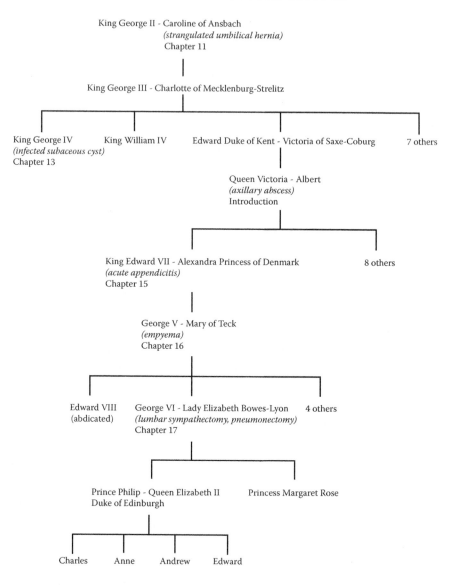

Figure 19.1 **The family tree of King George VI.**

So, in bringing this little volume to an end, I would like to recommend a study of the great operations of the past to our present young surgeons – on their shoulders fall the responsibilities of the next generation of 'historic operations'.